The International Behavioural and Social Sciences Library

SOCIAL SCIENCE AND GOVERNMENT

TAVISTOCK

The International Behavioural and Social Sciences Library

SOCIOLOGY & SOCIAL POLICY
In 10 Volumes

I Social Theory and Economic Change
Edited by Tom Burns and S B Saul

II Social Science and Government
Edited by A B Cherns, et al.

III The Use of Models in the Social Sciences
Edited by Lyndhurst Collins

IV Sociology and Development
Edited by Emanuel de Kadt and Gavin Williams

V Public Planning
J K Friend, et al.

VI Immigration and Social Policy in Britain
Catherine Jones

VII The Social Analysis of Class Structure
Edited by Frank Parkin

VIII The Rules of the Game
Edited by Teodor Shanin

IX Value Systems and Social Process
Geoffrey Vickers

X The Action-Image of Society
Alfred Willener

SOCIAL SCIENCE AND GOVERNMENT

Policies and Problems

EDITED BY A B CHERNS, R SINCLAIR
AND W I JENKINS

Routledge
Taylor & Francis Group
LONDON AND NEW YORK

First published in 1972 by
Tavistock Publications Limited

Reprinted in 2001 by
Routledge
2 Park Square, Milton Park, Abingdon, Oxon, OX14 4RN

Simultaneously published in the USA and Canada by Routledge
711 Third Avenue, New York, NY 10017

Transferred to Digital Printing 2007

First issued in paperback 2013

Routledge is an imprint of the Taylor & Francis Group, an informa business

The publishers have made every effort to contact authors/copyright holders of the works reprinted in the *International Behavioural and Social Sciences Library*. This has not been possible in every case, however, and we would welcome correspondence from those individuals/companies we have been unable to trace.

These reprints are taken from original copies of each book. In many cases the condition of these originals is not perfect. The publisher has gone to great lengths to ensure the quality of these reprints, but wishes to point out that certain characteristics of the original copies will, of necessity, be apparent in reprints thereof.

British Library Cataloguing in Publication Data
A CIP catalogue record for this book
is available from the British Library

Social Science and Government

ISBN 978-0-415-26496-9 (hbk)
ISBN 978-0-415-86907-2 (pbk)

Social Science and Government

Policies and Problems

Edited by

A. B. CHERNS

R. SINCLAIR

W. I. JENKINS

TAVISTOCK PUBLICATIONS

First published in 1972
by Tavistock Publications Limited
2 Park Square, Milton Park, Abingdon, Oxon, OX14 4RN
in 11 pt. Garamond, 1½ pt. leaded
by The Camelot Press Ltd, London and Southampton

The paper by Henri Mendras was written for the journal *Analyse et Prévision* (Paris), in which it was published in May 1968. Copyright SEDEIS.

SBN 422 73950 2

Proceedings of an
International Social Science Council Conference
on Social Science Policy
April 1970

Distributed in the USA by
HARPER & ROW PUBLISHERS, INC.
BARNES & NOBLE IMPORT DIVISION

Dedicated to Clemens Heller

Contents

Part 2 Aspects of Social Science Policy

Preface

The conference whose proceedings are reported in this volume was convened to discuss issues and problems concerned with the establishment of internal and external policies for the social sciences. The conference was sponsored and arranged through the auspices of the International Social Science Council (ISSC) who had identified the topic as one of importance that had been neglected in many national contexts by social scientists and governments alike. Many of the ideas and initiatives in this area sprang out of the interests of Clemens Heller (École practique des hautes études, Paris) who, together with Albert Cherns, was responsible for formulating the plans from which the conference developed.

The organization and co-ordination of the conference were carried out by the ISSC, and here particular note must be made of the efforts and work of Dr Samy Friedman, ISSC's Secretary General, and his staff in making the occasion the success it was. Thanks must also be given to Dr Harry Alpert, Director of the Division of Social Sciences, UNESCO, for his continuing help and interest in the project and to UNESCO in particular for financial assistance and for permission to reproduce several of the papers in the conference proceedings. Dr Geoffrey Roberts played an invaluable part in the preliminary preparations for the meeting, while Dr Elisabeth Crawford convened the Round Table on Research and Development Statistics. In conclusion, the editors owe a debt of gratitude to Mrs Gloria Brentnall for her skilful and patient work in preparing the manuscripts for publication.

Members of the conference

Dr Harry Alpert, Director, Department of Social Sciences, UNESCO

Dr Orville Brim Jr, President, Russell Sage Foundation, New York

Professor G. Carvalho, Universidade Federal de Minas Gerais, Brazil

M. M. B. Cazes, Commissariat Général au Plan, Paris

Professor A. B. Cherns, Department of Social Sciences, Loughborough University of Technology, UK

Dr Elisabeth Crawford, École pratique des hautes études, Paris

Dr Henning Friis, Director, Danish National Institute of Social Research, Copenhagen

Professor Sherwood Fox, Visiting Professor of Sociology, Sociological Institute, University of Copenhagen

Dr S. Friedman, Secretary General, International Social Science Council, Paris

Professor Dietrich Goldschmidt, Director, Institut für Bildungsforschung, Max-Planck-Gesellschaft, Berlin

Professor Sjoerd Groenmann, President, International Social Science Council, Paris, and Professor of Sociology, University of Utrecht, The Netherlands

Professor Clemens Heller, École pratique des hautes études, Paris

Mr M. P. Janosi, Ford Foundation, New York

Dr W. I. Jenkins, Department of Social Sciences, Loughborough University of Technology, UK

Dr H. M. Jolles, Professor of Sociology, Sociological Institute, University of Amsterdam

Professor Bertrand de Jouvenel, Faculty of Law and Economics, University of Paris

Mr Julian Knox, Adviser, Aide à tout Détresse, Paris

Professor L. Kredar, Secretary General, International Union of Anthropological and Ethnological Science, Department of Anthropology, Syracuse University, New York

Professor Paul Lazarsfeld, Department of Social Sciences, Columbia University, New York

M. Bernard-Pierre Lecuyer, Centre d'études sociologiques, Paris

M. P. Meluyn, ILO, Geneva

Professor Henri Mendras, Centre for Sociological Studies, University of Nanterre, France

Mr Jeremy Mitchell, Scientific Secretary, UK Social Science Research Council, London

Dr Geoffrey K. Roberts, Department of Social Sciences, Loughborough University of Technology, UK

Professor S. Rokkan, Professor of Sociology, University of Bergen, Norway, and Visiting Professor in Political Science, Yale University, New Haven, USA

M. Jean-Jacques Salamon, Directorate for Scientific Affairs, OECD, Paris

Mr Andrew Shonfield, Chairman, UK Social Science Research Council, London

Mrs Ruth Sinclair, Department of Social Sciences, Loughborough University of Technology, UK

Professor B. Suchodolski, Academy of Sciences, Warsaw, Poland

Professor J. Szczepanski, Institute of Philosophy and Sociology, Warsaw, Poland

Professor Einar Thorsrud, Work Research Institutes, Oslo, Norway

Professor Eric Trist, Wharton School of Finance and Commerce, University of Pennsylvania, Philadelphia, USA

M. Jean Viet, Services d'éxchange d'informations scientifiques, Paris

Professor A. T. M. Wilson, Professor of Organizational Behaviour, London Graduate School of Business Studies, London

PRESENTED PAPERS BUT WERE UNABLE TO ATTEND

Professor Yehezkel Dror, Faculty of Social Sciences, Hebrew University of Jerusalem, and RAND Corporation, USA

Dr Henry W. Riecken, President, US Social Science Research Council, Washington

Introduction

At a time when international conferences are counted by the hundred, no particular justification is needed for holding yet another. The rationale for such conferences is familiar enough and no one would be so churlish as to begrudge a few social scientists a week in Paris in the spring.

And of course each conference is unique; otherwise it would not be held. Furthermore while many international conferences are the first of their kind some inspire no successors and are thus the last as well as the first. So the fact that the first international conference on social science policy was held in Paris from 13 to 16 April 1970 is hardly headline news. Nevertheless that it was significant, even a portent, will have to emerge from the papers and the discussions.

One significant point, however, is implicit in holding the conference at all. In order to hold a conference about a topic, you do not necessarily have to obtain agreement that the name represents any reality, nor that its meaning is the same for all participants, although there are always tiresome people who may demand a definition. But you do have to obtain agreement that the topic is worth talking about, writing papers about, and going to some inconvenience for. Thus while it would be wrong to conclude that, because a conference was held on 'social science policy', a comprehensive social science policy actually exists anywhere or that the participants thought that it did, it would be right to conclude that they thought that the question of whether a social science policy existed was both meaningful and important; that the question of whether a social science policy or social science policies should exist was also important; and that they were highly concerned about what the content of such a policy should be and about the institutional framework for making and implementing social science policy. Strangely, institutions of this kind have been set up whose structure and functions would be summed up most economically by an outside observer in the phrase 'social science policy-making', yet without any mention in their charter, statutes, or whatever, of the phrase, or even of a suitably guarded synonym. It is broadly true to say that most countries and organizations have had no social science policy in a prospective sense, though their actions may cumulate to display a policy in retrospect.

PRE-HISTORY OF SOCIAL SCIENCE POLICY

The pre-history of social science policy like the pre-history of science policy antedates the arbitrary divisions of these and other branches of knowledge. Bacon, the favourite adopted ancestor of philosophers of science and proponents of science policy, distinguished between 'science' and 'arts' considering the former as knowledge and the latter as the use of knowledge, warning against 'the over-ready and peremptory reduction of knowledge into arts and methods; from which time commonly sciences receive small or no argumentation' (Bacon, *The Advancement of Learning*). The problem of 'pure' versus 'applied' remains with us.

Bacon also proposed a model for the organization of science in *The New Atlantis*, not neglecting the international character of the enterprise. Within this organization he posited roles with regard to the collection and collation of information, the design and execution of new experiments, and the utilization of knowledge from these to design yet further experiments and to formulate comprehensive and wide-ranging theory. In addition he identified the need for specialists to carry out these tasks. But of course the systematic use of the natural sciences in the service of the state was not to take place for a long time, and a similar development in the social sciences is just beginning.

THE PRESSURES: POLICY FOR, OR POLICY FOR USING?

The first modern example of such a systematic attempt is described by Gene Lyons (1969). It comes as a little of a surprise to find that the name associated with an attempt to mobilize the social sciences for an attack on the social problems confronting a country is that of President Herbert Hoover. In 1929 he set up the President's Research Committee on Social Trends with the remit 'to examine and to report upon recent social trends in the United States with a view to providing such a review as might supply a basis for the formulation of large national policies looking to the next phase in the nation's development'. The commission, which numbered many distinguished American social scientists, presented their interim conclusions in a document entitled *Recent Social Trends* (1933), which went largely unremarked in the turmoil of the 1930s. Interest in it has revived in the context of the current concern with 'social indicators'.

The most recent developments to have raised the issue of social science policy have been the more-or-less simultaneous growth of two pressures upon governments. The first has been the growth of expectations about the utilization of the social sciences in dealing with social and economic problems; the second has been the growth in the budgeting and manpower demands made by the social sciences. These two strands – policy for using the social sciences and policy for developing the social sciences – have become inseparable. One cannot talk sensibly about the amount of resources that *should be* devoted to the social sciences without raising the question of what the social sciences are *for*. Nevertheless many social scientists are anxious to apply themselves to the former question and becomingly reluctant to expose themselves by examining the latter question. Governments are prone to adopt the reverse order of priority. Whether explicit or not, claims made by social scientists for resources carry implications about the potential use to which social science is to be put. Our answers to questions of 'should' inevitably rest upon our systems of values, and claims imply values of some kind. For example, suppose we take the extreme position that the social sciences *should be* supported for their own sake and not for any contribution they may have the power to make towards solving problems. Such a claim rests upon the *value* of adding to knowledge or to the education of citizens. Apart from the fact that there is in such a claim no explicit basis for preferring social science to art, to sport, or to poetry in allocating resources, there is an appeal to a (presumably shared) value system, which considers pure knowledge as desirable and worthy of receiving support at the expense of some other activity. The unvoiced utility expectation is that the study of sociology or economics develops the intellect as poetry does our sensibilities and sport does our bodies. The problem of use has not been solved, it has just been ducked.

There is more than one reason why social scientists adopt an ambiguous attitude towards this question of use. First, there is of course the proper humility of the scientist, unwilling to make claims he fears he will be unable to redeem. Second, the social scientist cannot simultaneously claim support on the grounds of the usefulness of his work to the aims of government and arrogate to himself the choice of what work he will do; thus he fears loss of his freedom to pursue his own chosen line of research (one of the strands that go to make up the cherished cord of 'academic freedom'). Third, he mistrusts the governments to make the use he would wish of his work; if not the present government, then some possible future ones. Fourth, his position of 'critic' of society is weakened by his acceptance of the ends to which his contribution may be put. It would be idle to pretend that the essays in this book resolve the dilemma; at most they may help to clarify the issues and their consequences. They show that the basis upon which decisions can be made about the social sciences' share in resources is itself a question for social science research. Almost every discussion tends to take for granted that social science directed towards use will in fact be used. The conditions under which use is possible have scarcely been investigated. The kinds of use to which social science knowledge has been put have only sketchily been analysed. Yet the extent to which such knowledge can be used is fundamental to both sides of the argument – to the claim for support on the grounds of potential utility, and to the fears of misuse or use to ends unsanctioned by the social scientist. In discussion, Lazarsfeld called for a 'science of utilization'.

CULTURAL RELATIVITIES

A science of this kind would soon expose the intimate relationships between the development of the social sciences and their cultural, national, historical, and sociopolitical origins. Defining the social sciences sounds an arid, academic exercise; however, examining the different *de facto* definitions adopted in different countries or in the same country at different times is illuminating – this is particularly so of the national attitudes towards, and expectations from, them. If the actual subject-matter of economics is not greatly dissimilar in different countries this reflects less the certainties of economics than the shared use of conventions about the ways of relating the values of disparate items and about the relevance of certain kinds of indicators to the assessment of goal achievement. This is not quite the same thing as saying that the material goals of countries are similar while their social goals differ, though the two points are connected. Indeed the connection is an interactive one – the adoption of a mode of measuring has a considerable influence upon what will be selected to be measured and hence upon what will be regarded as having value.

The most topical instance of this point is the one repeatedly made concerning environmental pollution. The gross national product is increased by the expenditure incurred in creating pollution and by the cost of cleaning it up, and action incurring no expenditure, which prevents the pollution in the first place, adds nothing to the GNP. So long as an arbitrary selection of indicators is used for calculating GNP, increases in the GNP will fail to represent the true increments of welfare to society. The search for social indicators to correct imbalances of this nature is discussed in Chapter 4.

The content of the issues that will be regarded in any particular society as sociological or political or philosophical or psychological depends to a considerable extent on the ideological presuppositions of that society. To make an easy point, the 'problem' of poverty may present itself as a theological or a sociological or an economic problem depending both on prior beliefs about the 'meaning' of poverty and on the state of knowledge.

So long as poverty was believed to be divinely decreed, the problem was to determine its purpose; a search for means of eliminating it would appear blasphemous. On the other hand the comparatively sophisticated means of influencing economic activity available to governments, compared with the much cruder means available to them of producing changes in social attitudes and actions, have inclined them to perceive poverty primarily in economic terms, and only when economic development has still left a stubborn core of distress has the problem come to be perceived in more sociological terms. Thus the state of knowledge, the tools available, and the terms in which problems are perceived are inextricably intertwined; the content of any of the social sciences cannot be sensibly regarded as having definitive meaning outside its social context. Any attempts to develop policies for, or for the uses of, the social sciences must accommodate this fact.

It is at the same time one of the most pressing reasons why a policy for the social sciences *as a whole* is required rather than separate policies for the separate social sciences. Academic organization and the dynamics of the growth and development of disciplines tend to emphasize the differences among different disciplines; to arrogate issues to their subject-matter is somewhat arbitrary and is not identical across traditions or unchanging through time. Furthermore, as is brought out in the discussions, real-life social problems do not fall neatly into disciplinary divisions. As one of the contributors to the conference, Dr A. T. M. Wilson, is fond of quoting, 'God did not see fit to distribute problems in accordance with the titles of university chairs'.

HOW HOMOGENEOUS ARE THE SOCIAL SCIENCES?

That there are problems involved in treating the social sciences as a whole is brought out strongly by Andrew Shonfield. Many economists regard their own discipline as so much more 'advanced' than the other social sciences that co-operation with other social scientists is seen as unrewarding. This claim to relative 'advancement' rests very largely upon greater, more precise, and more sophisticated use of mathematical methods and techniques. To that extent it is well founded. It assumes, however, that there is only one way for a science to advance and it has exercised a distorting effect on neighbouring disciplines, some of whose practitioners have come to overvalue what is measurable and the attainment of means of measuring. The development of biology has not followed the course of development of physics, and the extent that the use made of mathematics in physics has been influential in biology has been not because biologists have imitated physicists but because some physicists have become interested in biological problems to which the techniques they had used in physics look applicable.

Fortunately the realization that what appear to be 'economic' problems are not solvable in economic terms is spreading. Gunnar Myrdal (1968) put it: economists are 'naïvely innocent of their own social determinants. This unawareness is reflected in their separation of economic from non-economic factors ... Economic models have come to stereotype this whole way of thinking ... and in turn have strongly influenced the plans and the discussion of planning for developments in the South Asian countries ... this particular type of model-thinking has systematically biased the planners' view of reality ... The economic models used in planning ... can be studied as manifestations of certain habits of thought and social pressures that result in biases. As such: the investigation is part of the sociology of knowledge.' Sir Alex Cairncross (1969), chief economic adviser to the British government, said even more bluntly, 'There are no economic problems, only problems.'

The need for associating economics with the other social sciences in policy formation, however well established, does not mean that there are no difficulties in the way of doing so. The special situation of economics is recognized more on the utilization side of policy than on the side concerned with policy for the development of, and allocation of resources to, the disciplines themselves. Such institutions as the American Council of Economic Advisors attest this, as does the widespread employment of economists in a professional capacity in government and other major institutions such as banks and insurance companies. Some other social scientists, sociologists for example, tend to see this model for their own discipline without an adequate examination of the experience of economists in professional and advisory capacities. Their existence is assumed as proof of their success; we have not sought to discover in what ways economists have been effective and what aspects of their knowledge and advice their employers have been able to utilize.

RELATIONSHIP TO SCIENCE POLICY

One of the major stimuli to the discussion of social science policy has been the development and growth on an international scale of science policy. It would be pointless to deny the element of me-too-ism, even a certain bandwaggon effect. But even without these the question of a social science policy was bound to follow in the wake of science policy. For one thing the demands that social scientists now make on national resources in a number of countries bears comparison with the demands made by the natural scientists some 20 years ago. It by no means follows that these demands will grow at the same rate or for the same reason, but their inherent tendency to grow is obvious and the need for a planned response to these demands becomes equally obvious. To the evident parallels between science policy and social science policy-making we need to add a consideration of their interrelationship.

In the first place the organizational development of the social sciences has not only paralleled, but has also to some extent been modelled on, organizational forms devised for the natural sciences. A notable example of this is the organization of research training. Certainly the need for such organizations has arisen out of developments within the social sciences, but the forms that they have then taken owe much to the example of the natural sciences. While it could be argued that organizational forms modelled on those devised for the natural sciences may be inappropriate to the social sciences, there seems no doubt that the adoption of such models has unquestionably influenced the way in which the social sciences have developed.

Another outcome has been the inclination of governments and administrators to perceive the social sciences as essentially little brothers of the natural sciences, bound to follow in their footsteps but stumbling because of their infancy. This conception, to which social scientists themselves have unfortunately contributed, may have done a good deal of damage. It should certainly put us on our guard against assuming too readily that what is good for the natural sciences is necessarily good for the social sciences.

The second respect in which science policy is related to social science is in regard to the shifting boundary between the natural and social science disciplines. The boundaries of disciplines are of course not immutable; part of the process of development of a discipline is in fact the advancing of its boundaries, sometimes at the expense of or encroachment upon the territory formerly claimed by other disciplines. New sub-disciplines or even disciplines may arise as techniques developed in one science become applicable to problems arising in another. People cross the boundary with their techniques. Thus we have comparatively recently witnessed repeated crossings of the boundaries between the physical and the life sciences and the recent emergence of biophysics. This kind of activity has been less significant either between life sciences and social sciences or between physical sciences and social sciences, but it has been occurring none the less. The boundaries between physiology and psychology have long been hazy; psychopharmacology has grown in this borderland. Likewise the boundaries between psychology and various engineering disciplines have become the territory of ergonomists. More recently still the development of general systems theory has been the umbrella under which sheltered trading of concepts and methods has taken place among engineering, the life sciences, and the social sciences.

Closely allied to this development is the coming together of social scientists and other scientists on problems that cannot be resolved by the exercise of one expertise alone. A good example is the current concern with the environment. Biologists, sociologists, engineers, economists, psychologists, and political scientists are all being brought into the attempts to assess the state of, and changes in, the environment and its effects on social life and human life chances. In one particular aspect, the built environment, psychologists, sociologists, economists, and engineers and architects have been learning to work together. Technological assessment and technological forecasting are rapidly developing as foci of this kind of multidisciplinary activity. These not only bind social and other scientists together in a way that requires the modification of institutional forms to accommodate their joint endeavours, they are themselves critical issues in science policy.

Finally, the social sciences along with the natural sciences form the most rapidly growing of all industries—the knowledge industry. The same problems of information storage and retrieval face both. Governments are bound to evolve policies for this industry and these could, without adequate analysis of the specific needs and problems of utilization of the social sciences, take the form of a maladaptive application of the principles of science policy.

We must foresee a growing interest in the social sciences on the part of organs, both national and international, whose primary mission is science policy. Our consideration of what is and what is not desirable, what is and what is not practicable, will have to comprehend this development.

In this light we need to look closely at the organs of social science policy that exist or are coming into existence. We note that where research councils are the preferred method for the natural sciences, social science research councils with broadly similar remits have been, or are being, created. Where national Academies of Science serve as science policy-making bodies, divisions or sections of social sciences exist within them. To a considerable extent, then, social science policies are being created in the image of science policies whether this is truly appropriate or not.

In a comprehensive review of the situation in the United States Riecken (Chapter 9) shows how the pluralistic model of the organization of scientific research in his country is parelleled, even exceeded, by the pluralism of support for the social sciences. The United States model is unique and likely to remain so. One could argue that if a country treats the social sciences in a way broadly similar to that in which it treats the natural sciences, this is no more than a demonstration of the fact that particular societies are likely to evolve similar methods for dealing with similar problems. This is true but begs the question whether the problems are truly similar or whether the existence of a particular method has pre-empted the evolution of other methods by its very existence, and in the absence of any critical examination of its aptness.

In yet another way we can perceive a parallel between the problems of science policy and those of social science policy. Suspicious of the continued growth of science at a rate exceeding that of the economy as a whole, and critical of the uses to which science has been put, many have been questioning whether scientists are the right people to be advising governments on their science policies. Precisely the same question may be asked of us. Are social scientists specially qualified to tender advice to governments and other users on their social science policies?

SOCIAL SCIENTISTS AS POLICY-MAKERS

It is obvious that social scientists having a particular interest in the allocation of funds to their disciplines are likely to be drawn into overstating their case if their role is that of mendicant or even of advocate. But who is to say that it is overstated, who is competent to judge? Of course making judgements upon issues in which they are inexpert is the daily lot of the politician and of the generalist administrator. Lacking any other basis for judgement he may resort to precedent or to compromise, neither in themselves necessarily the wrong guide but sometimes producing unfortunate, unfair, even occasionally disastrous results. He may resort to asking his specialist adviser who is trained to perform the role of counter-advocate. This may even go so far as the staging of a confrontation with something of a courtroom atmosphere, with the administrator as the judge above the battle. If this appears to us as social scientists to be unsatisfactory, we are faced with proposing something better which does not at the same time appear to arrogate to ourselves the functions of judges in our own cause.

We may start with an examination of our own special capacities. We may with some justice claim that we are better fitted than anyone else to understand and assess the capabilities of the social sciences, to advise on what they are likely to be able to do in the present state of knowledge. This claim can, however, only be fully validated if we are prepared to undertake what in the past we have not done, a continuously updated review of both the state of knowledge and the state of the art of application. There is of course as always the other side of the balance. To a social-science-performing capability must be added a social-science-utilizing capability which is a function of the administration itself. In the course of the discussions reported in this book there was agreement that we need to develop this capability and that this was itself an important area of social science activity. Thus another special function of the social scientist in his advisory role is the assessment and upgrading of the social-science-utilizing capability of the organization he is advising.

This is an important point. While numerous organizations such as government departments have appointed advisory committees or councils of social scientists to recommend to them the social science research they should undertake or sponsor, few if any have asked their committee to examine their capability to use the research. Nor have such committees pressed this issue themselves, either because they have not regarded it as within their province or, more culpably, because they are themselves totally unaware of the need. Too few social scientists have served on both sides of the utilization fence; if more were to do so we could expect a higher level of sophistication and understanding of the problems.

We are coming close to saying that eminence in research or teaching in a social science does not *ipso facto* equip a person with the knowledge needed to advise governments or other organizations on their social science policy. Some knowledge of a critically relevant nature is possessed by others perhaps themselves less eminent; some vital knowledge just does not exist. The former problem can be resolved by a suitable mix of experience in an advisory body; the latter cannot, and can be dealt with only by more study. Among the topics in need of more research are (a) the dynamics of the development of the social sciences, (b) the effects of attempts to apply social science knowledge and research, and (c) the policy process itself.

(a) The dynamics of development of the social sciences

What are the appropriate institutional frameworks for maximizing the advance of knowledge in the social sciences? It is usually tacitly assumed that this advance is in the good hands of university departments and a few research institutes. Trist indicates in his paper (Chapter 6) that this is too simple a notion. The most effective activity mix for different purposes is a matter for study and planning; Trist proposes a useful paradigm for analysis. Institution-building is an essential aspect of social science policy; we are only just beginning to learn something systematic about its nature and process.

(b) The effects of applying social science knowledge and research

As social scientists we know a good deal about social and organizational change. Certainly we know enough to warn us that these are diachronic processes and that any before-after comparison entails arbitrary divisions of time. We also know that many such comparisons are invalidated by insufficient knowledge of the 'before' condition, that the changes have already begun, or been foreshadowed, before monitoring has started. We know that a true monitoring is possible only if we are in a position to establish the necessary indicators early enough for a reliable pre-change series of readings to be obtained. But this is only conceivable where a relatively long-term engagement of social scientists with the institution concerned has been established. Just because these conditions are so infrequently met we have very few reliable studies of the effects of application. Here the policy and the need for adequate knowledge on which to base the policy are intertwined. First we must have the policy of long-term engagement; then we can have knowledge about the effects of applying social science; finally we can use that knowledge to recommend policy.

(c) The policy process

This usefully illustrates the essentially serial nature of policy-making and brings us to the third point: knowledge about the policy process itself. Thorsrud in his paper (Chapter 3) presented an insight into this that was fresh to many of his hearers. He demonstrated that the role of the social scientist in policy-making about research and its utilization was a continuous one, taking different forms at different points in the process. He argued cogently that we are still inadequately informed about the process, and that without more substantive knowledge we cannot plan the most effective intervention into it.

Mendras (Chapter 7) provided a fascinating insight into the vagaries that influence the acceptance or rejection of ideas deriving from the social sciences. The validity of the ideas can be of less importance than the state of receptiveness of the politician or administrator, whose receptiveness is influenced by his particular current preoccupations as much as by long-term ideological considerations.

This raises not only disturbing questions about the potential misuse of good social science and the potential use of bad social science but also fundamental questions about the points of leverage in a system – where will an intervention be likely to have most effect? To some extent this brings us back to Thorsrud's discussion of the policy-making processes; without adequate knowledge of these the points or planes of leverage cannot be forecast.

Inevitably one finds discussion of policy focusing on the actions of governments and government agencies. The very notion of a social science policy presupposes the existence of a single decision-making body whose decisions are or can be effective – in a word that somebody is in control. We need occasionally, perhaps frequently, to be reminded that many organizations and many individuals are taking decisions about matters within their province which are, or imply, policy decisions about the social sciences. When a university senate votes to increase the enrolments of students of economics or to create a chair in sociology, or to reject a proposal for a post-graduate course in social ecology, it is taking decisions that affect the social science capability of that university and also of the wider community. When the trustees of a powerful foundation vote to commit resources to the study of race relations or to terminate its programme for the study of educationally backward children, they are taking possibly quite far-reaching decisions about both social science capability and social-science-utilizing capabilities. When I decide to devote some thought and effort to the question of social science policy, I am, I hope, taking a decision that may have some eventual impact on the making of social science policy.

Riecken (Chapter 9) shows how social science policy in the United States can have little meaning except as a summation or product of the decisions made by an unknown, virtually unknowable, number of institutions, organizations, and individuals. This is a fact not a lament; few people in the United States would want it to be otherwise. But this does not mean that anarchy must reign. Nor, on the other hand, does it imply that the government must in some way try to co-ordinate all these disparate activities. What is implied is that policy-makers need to take into account the existence of plural independent sources of policy; that they need to know the nature of the system with which they are concerned. For they too wish their own policies to have maximum impact and must therefore be concerned with the points of leverage to which they have access. For example, the National Science Foundation has chosen as such a point the standard of social science teaching in some of the less well-provided universities and colleges. The Federal writ does not run in the field of education, which is a state or private preserve, but using the device of training fellowships and summer courses it has intervened effectively. A pluralist system does not necessarily defeat or hinder the making or implementation of policy; it may indeed assist it through a multiplier or an amplifier effect. Social scientists need to provide policy-makers and themselves with utilizable models of the system they inhabit.

Thorsrud (Chapter 3) points out that policy for utilization of the social sciences is not a monopoly of governments. The Norwegian experiments in industrial democracy can teach many lessons and not the least of these is the concept of the 'learning system'. The policy-making system itself needs to be able to learn, to adopt modifications on the basis of its own built-in feedback. We are a long way from such a system, but the Norwegian experiments at least point the road.

Not the least of the complications surrounding the issue of social science policy is that it is in some ways an arbitrary abstraction. There are comparatively few decisions that could be regarded as matters of social science policy and of no other kind of policy. Goldschmidt (Chapter 5) shows that social science manpower is also an aspect of educational policy; and a very considerable proportion of all social science policy issues are also issues of educational policies. Similarly, decisions about the financing of social science research are part of overall government fiscal and monetary policy; likewise decisions about sponsoring research of an 'applied' nature; even more, policies concerning the utilization of social science research are also decisions about the substantive policy field with which the research is concerned. For example, a decision to establish a division of research and planning in a department of housing is equally a decision in the field of housing policy and in social science policy. When the system with which we are dealing appears so closely interrelated with other systems that we are obliged to direct our attention to a super-system embracing them, we need, as well as policies, policies about how policies should be made; what Dror has called 'meta-policies' (Chapter 12).

THE INTERNATIONAL NATURE OF THE SOCIAL SCIENCES

The most significant meta-system is the international one. The knowledge industry knows no national boundaries. Policy decisions in the field of the social sciences that are made in one country very soon affect another. First, they may influence the movement of social scientists from one country to another; second, they serve as precedents or signposts to social scientists; third, the output of any research stimulated or sponsored by the particular policy will be published and read in other countries, discussed at international conferences, and become part of the stock of knowledge of the entire international social science community. Clearly not all areas of social sciences are equally international in character. Macro-economics and experimental psychology are relatively non-culturally specific; community studies may be very culturally specific indeed and generate little of a more widely applicable nature than the methods of inquiry used. One of the important questions remains: just how culture-bound is any particular micro-level finding? This question is fundamental both to the status of the finding itself and to its practical implications. It has in the past been too readily assumed that findings from American industrial studies would prove applicable in, for example, India. Only the failures of hopeful schemes have drawn our attention to social and cultural factors at a level at which they were formerly ignored or unsuspected. We are now even asking questions about the effect of a laboratory 'culture' on the psychological experiment conducted with single human subjects.

The supra-national character of the social science enterprise is not an attic storey superimposed on a complete building: it is a basic part of the structure and cannot be ignored in any effective national policy-making for the social sciences. In turn this places what amounts virtually to an obligation on international bodies concerned with the social sciences to evolve not only policies for their own social science activities but a meta-policy for national social science policy-making. This point has been tacitly accepted, if not explicitly and in full, by the International Social Science Council (ISSC) which has, as an outcome of the conference reported in this book, established a committee on social science policy.

THE ROLE OF INTERNATIONAL BODIES

One field in which it can be said international bodies have taken a policy lead is the application of social sciences to the congeries of problems subsumed under the heading of 'development'. UNESCO in particular has been vigorously active in sponsoring conferences, research, and experiments in the field of development and, of course, has now a long history of efforts to promote social science capabilities in developing countries. Some of the assumptions that were made in the early stages of these efforts have now been modified as a result of experience; in fact a good deal has been learned about the problems of 'implantation'. Even more is now known about the problems of applying the social sciences to the field of economic development; the early enthusiasm, even naïvety, which too readily assumed that economic development was a matter of applied economics, has been replaced by a sober estimate of the tasks facing social scientists of all varieties. To some degree this is taking the form of a concern with the social-science-utilizing capability of developing countries as well as with their social science capability. As usual, problem-solving capacity is least where problems are greatest – particularly when part of the problem is the lack of problem-solving capacity – a meta-problem indeed! The greatest need for social science is met by those countries whose own supply of social scientists is least, whose social scientists are least likely to want to work in 'applied' fields of low prestige, and whose social scientists are most likely to emigrate. Plugging the dyke with short-term attachments from abroad has yielded often little more than minor relief and has sometimes brought major problems of its own.

In contrast to policies for national social science policy-making – the meta-policy of the international body – this area of social science and development is one where international bodies alone can have an effective substantive policy, concerning as it does the international movement of social science and social scientists and the development of trans-national, cross-cultural knowledge and expertise. But this in turn must form one of the environmental factors to be taken into account in national social science policy-making. International bodies themselves have the resources neither of people nor of material to carry out a policy of this nature. Its effectiveness depends upon the co-operation of national bodies and implies that this co-operation is a part of the national social science policy. UNESCO, ISSC, and other international bodies which have concerned themselves with the social sciences have been in the social science policy game all along; the national bodies whose co-operation was required were, and are, often not. One of the many problems that UNESCO faces is the fact that its own policy-ratifying body consists of delegations appointed by national governments that may or may not contain social scientists and whose social science members may or may not be representative of national social science policy-making bodies. This issue in itself may prove crucial in any attempt by UNESCO to develop an international social science policy.

The role of the International Social Science Council is both hopeful and ambiguous. It is hopeful because it has been the first to sponsor study of the nature of social science policy, the issues involved in it, and the problems facing its evolution. It has sponsored a conference devoted to its discussion and demonstrated the interest in many countries in the topic. Its role is ambiguous because its own structure rests on international associations representing individual social science disciplines. This provides a clear enough charter to assist in evolving policies *for* the social sciences, but does not provide a warrant to evolve policies *for the use of* the social sciences. As we have discussed earlier the one is probably impossible, even meaningless, without the other. The evolution of a function, other than purely the sponsorship of research in the field of social science policy, will depend upon evolution of its structure. For the time being the ISSC has probably advanced as far as it can; its new committee has an important, even crucial. task.

EVALUATION

In a book that reports the proceedings of a conference some attempt ought to be made to evaluate its success. This is not an easy task as the conference was not oriented towards conclusions or problem-solving. Essentially its aims were: first, to obtain some idea of the extent of interest in the topic; second, to take stock of the state of the knowledge about social science policy; third, to examine the comparability of experiences and problems across national boundaries and systems. The scholars invited to the conference were not in any sense representatives of national bodies, nor were they necessarily in positions concerned with policy-making, although some clearly were. At this stage we were aiming to bring together people who were studying and had studied these topics and problems. It was fortunate indeed that we were able to number among us people with responsibility in this field who could deepen the perceptions of others about the environment in which policy-making has to take place.

Its success must be judged by the reader of the papers and discussions that follow. What I believe is most striking is the degree of consensus about what issues were important and the extent to which certain themes constantly recurred. In a conference in which are discussed the uses to which social science research is to be put, the cross-cultural links required, the relationships between national and international bodies, and so on, a number of spectres hover. Camelot is a name that can still evoke a *frisson* in a sensitive hearer. The ethical problem may be there in a form unrecognized until assumptions are probed. The defenders of the value-free social science thesis have suffered many recent defeats and with each one the ideological assumptions implicit in research and even in its methodology are exposed. This exposure makes for better social science so long as it is not so exaggerated as to cast doubt on the validity of the social sciences as analytical tools. But it suggests the existence of ethical problems where formerly they had not been perceived. Yet such problems are not totally new, and again we may turn to Bacon for a long-standing but accurate portrayal of this dilemma: 'For the honest and just bounds of observation by one person on another extend no further but to understand him sufficiently not to give him offence, or whereby to be able to give him faithful counsel or whereby to stand upon reasonable guard or caution in respect of man's self' (Bacon, *The New Atlantis*). Hence with regard to ethics and to other topics, there seems little doubt that further study of social science policy will increase our awareness of some of the subtle implications of policies we take for granted.

It would not be rash to conclude that the conference demonstrated that the similarities in the problems faced in different countries were greater than the differences. In addition it appeared that the participants learned enough from one another to wish to continue to exchange experience, knowledge, and views. Last, the feeling of optimism generated in the conference discussions gave the ISSC the confidence needed to advance into the field. The optimism was for the possibilities for systematic examination of the multifarious topics making up 'social science policy' as an area for research, and about the timeliness of such examination. The need is there and growing, the endeavour has begun.

A. B. C.

References

BACON, FRANCIS, *The Advancement of Learning* and *The New Atlantis*. Oxford University Press, London, 1938.

CAIRNCROSS, A., The Managed Economy. *The Advancement of Science* **26**: pp. 64–74, 1969–70.

LYONS, G., *The Uneasy Partnership: Social Science and the Federal Government in the Twentieth Century*. Russell Sage Foundation, New York, 1969.

MYRDAL, G., *Asian Drama*, Vol. III, pp. 1942–3. Pantheon, New York, 1968.

President's Research Committee on Social Trends, *Recent Social Trends*. McGraw-Hill, New York, 1933.

Part 1
Social Science as a Policy Area

1 The functions and roles of the social sciences

Bertrand de Jouvenel

The question of what the 'appropriate' role of the social scientist might be in society at large, particularly as concerns the potential applicability of social science knowledge to topics defined as 'recognized problems', is one that has received a great deal of attention. Unfortunately much of this attention has remained at the level of polemic and is exemplified by two opposed stances: that which argues for the isolation of research as necessary for the development of social science theory, as against that which advocates the inescapable necessity of the social sciences advancing only through a direct involvement with discrete problems.

Many difficulties in the debate on these issues appear to arise from false analogies between the social sciences and the natural sciences – the sciences of man and the sciences of matter as Bertrand de Jouvenel terms them in his opening address. In this address de Jouvenel points to two major distinctions between the areas of social science and natural science – differences in knowledge and differences in thinking. Linked with differences in knowledge is the error of building repetitive models in the social sciences, i.e. models that have failed to take account of the phenomena of change; differences in thought mean that in many cases the aggregation of human actions is inadequate to provide a theoretical explanation for social behaviour. De Jouvenel by no means rejects the utility of quantitative measurement but does blame an over-emphasis on quantification for an intellectual conservatism in social science. The need as he sees it is not only to explain behaviour in a *post hoc* fashion by using aggregation as evidence, but to achieve a perspective whereby change can be anticipated.

Bertrand de Jouvenel is an economist whose studies and writings over forty years have dealt not only with economics but also with politics, political philosophy, and, recently, with the wider interdisciplinary area of future studies. At present a professor in the University of Paris, de Jouvenel is also director of the Institute SÉDÉIS and editor of the publication *Analyse et Prévision,* which encompasses the series 'Études futuribles'. He has since 1930 published many books and articles. His most recent volume, linked with his current leading interest in 'futures', is *The L'Art de la conjecture* (1964).

The place of science in society has grown enormously in the course of the last generation, whether growth is measured in terms of inputs or in terms of status. Indeed the status now achieved by science has been compared with that once enjoyed by religion. Laboratories invite the same awed reverence as did monasteries, and the endowment of research has become as much a social imperative as was the endowment of prayer.

Within this prestigious scientific establishment (Price, 1965), the social sciences have a minor and insecure standing: scientists have been reluctant to admit them into the scientific community, nor does the public trust them as it does the natural sciences.[1]

This inferiority of esteem in which the social sciences are held contrasts not only with their seniority but also with the urgently felt need for wise counsel in human affairs. This has been a century of total wars, totalitarian governments, and genocide. This is a world where most governments are born of violence or maintain themselves by coercion, and where even the most fortunate countries are plagued by the rise of criminality and the fanning of domestic differences into conflicts.

Therefore a moral obligation falls upon social scientists to guide their fellows to more amicable relations for the common good. It is not enough that they seek knowledge for itself, they must be prepared to apply it themselves.[2]

In my opinion consideration of the problem of beneficial performance by the social sciences requires some preliminary overview of the environment within which and upon which they have to operate. An overview is, of necessity, simplistic. But, as it haunts my mind and colours my perception of the subject, honesty calls for its statement.

A SOCIETY SHAPED BY MASTERY OF MATTER

I have alluded to the seniority of the social sciences. Indeed other fields of knowledge were hardly opened when problems of society, of conflict resolution and human excellence, were deeply discussed in Greece. But the society we live in has not been shaped by a successive development of such concerns. It has arisen from an utterly different source.

In fact our civilization, as it stands in the more advanced countries, is the daughter of the technologies and sciences of matter. (Technologies figure first since to a large degree they preceded the involvement of science.) It seems essential to dwell upon this point because from such fostering arise the features, concrete, psychological, and even intellectual, of the environment within and upon which we must operate.

All civilizations previous to our own were reared upon hegemonic symbiosis: our dominant association with plant and animal life. Not only did plant and animal life provide us with food as they had done from the beginning and still do, but it was from immediate products of life that we drew the great bulk of our raw materials, flax, wool, leather, and above all wood. Animals were our machines for transport and pulling, we had few other machines and little other auxiliary energy.

Going back only three centuries, it is striking to find how large was the use we made of diverse forms of life and their products, how narrow was the use we made of matter, lifeless and not proceeding immediately from life.

Associated logically with this scantiness of use was our scantiness of knowledge. While aware of the great diversity of the forms of life, we were extremely ignorant of the great diversity of the structures of matter and of the various properties attached thereto.

Fantastic progress in the understanding and handling of matter has made the modal way of life in the advanced countries of today utterly different from what it was three centuries ago.[3] As the present is an incomparably easier and larger way of life, it is small wonder that we should honour the sciences and technologies that have proved the fount of this improvement and which, moreover, promise ever further improvement. Rightly earned therefore is the primacy granted to the sciences of matter. The only discipline that ranks with them in the new Olympus is medicine, from which we expect long life. Its progress however has been very dependent upon that of physics and chemistry.

Because of this exalted standing of the sciences of matter, it is natural that the social sciences should tend to take them as a model.

But there are great obstacles to making knowledge of society in the image of knowledge of matter, and some serious objections to drawing our inspiration from the latter.

DIFFERENCES IN KNOWLEDGE

It is commonly granted that our knowledge of society is less than our knowledge of matter. Our attention will focus upon differences in kind.

Consider the penetrating knowledge our chemists have acquired of the constitution of petroleum, and, to be more specific, of Persian and Iraqi petroleum. What they now know so well is that selfsame naphtha which Pliny mentioned, and of which he stated that 'between Persia and Babylon' there were some fifteen places where its outpouring kept up a ceaseless torch of flames. So here the progress of knowledge is a deep delving into a structure which for some time existed, awaiting our understanding.

Or again let us consider the constitution of atoms, and, to be more specific, of Uranium 235. The structure into which the inquiring mind has so recently achieved penetration has been in existence for millions of years.

Thus the progress of knowledge in the sciences of matter is an ever deeper penetration of the mind into structures unchanged, of which our seekers make successive representative models, ever more adequate.

In contrast, social scientists of our day address themselves to swiftly changing structures. Previous representative models have therefore to be discarded by social scientists, not, as was the case with physical scientists, because these models were inadequate representations of what is, but because they were representations of what is no more. Instead of increasing their mental grasp of states of things that await investigation, they must keep pace with states of affairs that are flowing away.

Even the most elementary social structure, the household, changes, but much less than larger structures; New York City is assuredly not a City in the Aristotelean sense – implying the possibility of frequent assemblies of citizens to make their collective decisions. In the course of a few generations enormous new bodies, the giant corporations, for example, have appeared on the social scene. The mind boggles in seeking to imagine any analogical transformations in the solar or galactic system.

Ongoing metamorphosis makes it very difficult to build an edifice of trustworthy affirmations, such as we have in the physical sciences. Montesquieu (1748) sought the natural laws of society and opened his study with this statement: 'Laws in their widest acceptance are the necessary relations which derive from the nature of things'. But it was then in the nature of things, in the economic realm, that any bulky commerce was bound to the sea or waterways; in the political realm, that a speaker could address no more than the few thousand assembled in a public place, that news travelled only at the speed of sail or horse, that a ruler's vision of the provinces and foreign parts was made up of unequally lagged information.

Just a hundred years separate the *Communist Manifesto* (Marx & Engels, 1848) from *The Spirit of the Laws*: a century when social transformism is the dominant theme. This is indeed the core of Rousseau's work: he might be called the first of the social evolutionists, and the reaction to his pamphlets served to gel awareness of this phenomenon and to rally enthusiasm for it. Turgot and Bentham are of course positive evolutionists, and the accent becomes one of unbounded enthusiasm in Condorcet, Saint Simon, Comte, whose intellectual tone is akin to that of Beethoven's symphonies. Tocqueville must of course be mentioned. Hegel and Marx add a dialectical twist. It seems unquestionable that social transformism preceded and prepared the transformation of species.

It seems somewhat strange that while the chief social thinkers concentrated on change, neither political science nor economics did. In both these disciplines, right up to the First World War and somewhat beyond, theoretical work consisted mainly in developing the logical consequences of premises laid down in the eighteenth century.

Political science was addicted to Constitutionalism, economics to General Equilibrium, that is to static models. Constitutionalists took no notice of the fact that the typical citizen had ceased to be an independent operator, they did not face the fact that elected representatives were not competent in the more diverse problems accruing to government. General Equilibrium theorists took no notice of the ever-increasing importance of corporations, and in their perfect competition there was no room for capital accumulation from cash-flow. I find it telling that the intention of praising Walras 'highly' has led to calling him 'the Newton of Economics', as if there was some similarity between the changing social system and the solar system; most puzzling is that this form of praise should have been used by Samuelson.

It seems to me that it is only since the Second World War that the attention of the social scientist has been addressed mainly to change – going under the names of growth and development. This has been due in part, and mainly for economics, to the combined impressions made by the Great Depression and the Soviet Five Year Plans, but to a far greater degree and more generally to the notice taken of 'underdevelopment'.

DIFFERENCES IN THINKING

In the previous epoch of the social sciences, there was a pervasive influence of geometric ways of thinking. It is only in the more recent epoch that ways of thinking learned from the sciences of nature have been embraced with enthusiasm.

The very terms growth and development denote a reference to living organisms: the comparison of society with an organism was of course the great theme of Durkheim, and, before him, of Thomas Huxley. While there may be some uses for this analogy, carefully handled, it is undoubtedly bad and misleading to assume that each and every society is just the same organism at different degrees of development: as Chesterton would say, it is wrong to regard a lamb as an underdeveloped tiger – an image which incidentally leads us to stress that every organism has its appointed *terminus ad quem*, which is not the case with societies, and the present lamb may evolve into something better than either a sheep or a tiger.

It is, however, only in more general terms that the social sciences refer to the sciences of life: their methods have been derived from the sciences of matter.

Knowledge of the different forms of matter is basically knowledge of their properties, according to which they respond to different contacts or treatments. Forms of matter are wholly *lawful* objects, whereby I mean that objects of a given category cannot fail to respond all in the same way and always in the same way to the same contact or treatment. If sulphur fails to turn into sulphuric acid, then it is not sulphur: but shall we say that if a dog fails to respond to the whistle, then it is not a dog? As we move from forms of matter to higher and higher forms of life, we encounter increasingly irregular forms of behaviour.

How then can we apply in the social sciences the ways of thinking developed in the sciences of matter, which we have come to equate with the scientific method? There is safety in numbers: aggregate behaviour of sets or subsets offers a reassuring consistency and allows us to tie it by regular relationships with other factors. This practice has been developed with considerable success in economics, where indeed Tinbergen, as early as 1938, built an overall model of the economy consisting in a system of equations tying together a diversity of variables each representative of an aspect of aggregate behaviour. In this vision each of several aspects of behaviour, pertaining to overlapping sets of actors, is, so to speak, 'objectified'.

While economists could find regularity of response (*lawfulness* in the sense indicated above) only at a certain level of aggregation, it was comforting to them to learn that physicists discovered *unlawfulness* by reaching down well beneath the level at which forms of matter had been previously apprehended. However I cannot identify the individuality of human actions that depart from the average with the randomness of Brownian motion. On the one hand we are dealing with randomness and entropy, on the other with liberty that can be conducive to change.

And indeed here myths come to mind, which put chaos at the beginning of things, then order coming out of chaos, and then initiative with its attendant uncertainties. But let us leave this suggestion for further consideration.

We must go on from economics to other social sciences where the same effort has been made to find *lawfulness* at the level of some aggregates. Thus political scientists have sought to tie the aggregates of voting behaviour to social status: they have met with incomplete success. But political science has also shown that quite small groups of extreme militancy can, at times, play a decisive part: thus Communist power was installed in Russia by a tiny group; nor was the group that installed Fascism in Italy a large one. Political scientists have not found it possible to correlate the make-up of such groups with any factors of social status.

Turning now to sociology, we must hail Quételet as the first master of the scientific approach (1835). He set two problems: what are the determinants of the proportion of births, what are the determinants of the frequency of crimes of violence? The first falls to the demographers, and I am inadequately informed about their progress; the second falls to sociologists, and it is well known that this problem has not been solved.

The efforts to tie together by regular relationships various concrete aspects of social life are very worth while and have brought important results. Far be it from me to question the value of their pursuit. But we should not be surprised to find them inadequate in many cases. The phenomenon of consciousness increases in importance as we rise in the forms of animal life up to man. Men use their capacity to act, not in response to their 'objective' environment, in which case their actions would be explainable and predictable on an 'objective basis', but in response to their perception and appraisal of the environment, which is individual, more so and of more consequence in the case of different aspects.

No one would deny the following formulation: 'A person's values and other psychological predispositions direct his attention selectively to certain features of his milieu, and he interprets what he selectively perceives in the light of conscious memories and subjectively stored experience' (Sprout, 1965). But however excellent the statement, it can still be used to drive back the singularity of perception and appraisal into the fold of determination by objective circumstances though now diachronic, not synchronic. 'Many Americans are Catholics, being of Irish or Italian descent' or 'Germans are fearful of inflation, having experienced it under its galloping form' – here are trivial statements that refer a present feature of a psychological nature back to past concrete circumstances. And it is of course of immense importance to take into account differences of background.

But no combination of past and present circumstances will explain the birth of a new outlook, nor do we know of any way to explain, let alone predict, it. All we can do is to be attentive to its manifestations in words and deeds. And it is here that excessive reliance upon statistics may defeat us, since, by definition, views and behaviour that are original have no immediate weight in aggregates.

STATISTICS

Because I do not want my position on quantitative measurement to be mistaken, I must inject a personal note.

All my life I have been an ardent user of statistics:[4] so much do I prize them that, teaching a course on Society, I opened it with a lengthy historical account of the collection of figures, stressing that our morphological knowledge of society depends upon our wealth of collected figures.

However, statistics are, as the word (coined in 1746) indicates, descriptions of states. Recent statistics describe a 'present' (recent) state. Historical series make it possible to establish correlations between past changes. Thus statistics inform us as to what is or has been visible, and indeed as to what has been, previously to the present, of sufficient interest to be reported; and of course the collection of figures was begun to serve the military and fiscal needs of government.

As statistics, by definition, can but describe the past, and by nature stem from past concerns, we should not overestimate their value for drawing our attention to problems of the future. It is not statistics that give us warning of traffic congestion as a problem of the future, but the other way round: it is present awareness of traffic congestion that has given rise to projections of past trends, reinforcing concern by pointing to the worsening of an already present evil (Buchanan, 1963).

If environmental problems have now been declared the theme of the seventies, this is certainly not due to statistics, since there were, until alarm spread, no statistics about damage to environment. Deterioration of the environment has never figured in National Accounts, a point I have repeatedly complained about in my fifteen years' service on France's Commission of National Accounts. But of course it could not figure since National Accounts are about the structure of relations between men, marked by financial transactions, and our collective transactions with nature are not of that character. Here we have an instance of a systems analysis that represents only part of reality and thereby constitutes an obstacle to considering what its conceptualization has omitted.

From this instance, several lessons can be drawn: first, what is now recognized as an important problem of the future was not and could not be read out of statistics, which did not exist; second, the recognition of the problem must falsify to some extent projections of the economy made before such recognition, because the cost of clean air must come at the expense of other things, and, being a little more analytical, technological coefficients must be changed, as the nature of some inputs has to be altered to impede some noxious outputs; and, third, a new problem arises: what sort of trade-off shall in fact take place between the impatient demand for individual 'goods' and the alleviation of collective 'bads'; how willingly, for instance, will people accept more costly or less powerful cars which would be non-polluting; or again, at the level of government expenditure, what will be the trade-off between expenditures addressed to our national basis, and expenditures addressed to ghetto populations?[5]

Or to take another instance, the most careful study of past correlations could not predict, and cannot explain, the great upsurge of student militancy that travelled out from Berkeley and reached such astounding importance in Europe in 1968.

The point I wish to make here is that the social sciences have proved far too conservative intellectually. I wonder whether this is not due in part to a deliberate imitation of the physical sciences, implying however a misunderstanding of their true character. Michael Polanyi wrote:

> Scientists – that is, creative scientists – spend their lives in trying to guess right. They are sustained and guided therein by their heuristic passion. We call their work creative because it changes the world as we see it. . . . Major discoveries change our interpretative framework. Hence it is logically impossible to arrive at these by the continued application of our previous interpretative framework (Polanyi, 1958).

Now if we start with the last sentence, we find that it stresses discontinuity in science, and that clinging to a given interpretative framework cannot lead to discovery and would impede its reception. Working upwards, we find discovery equated with 'changing the world as we see it'.

Here arises a point of major interest. 'Changing the world as we see it' may be occasionally the work of some major social thinker, but mainly it is an ongoing phenomenon, occurring outside our professional circles, in some minds and spreading to others. Granted that it is so and that it affects behaviour, then the social scientist's guessing is about such ongoing or forthcoming changes of outlook.

This would be a foresight of how people may come to see. However excessive such an ambition, at least a concern of this nature would shift our attention somewhat from the reassuring lawfulness of averages to those small beginnings, of which some will come to nothing and others will have great momentum.

Notes

[1] This reluctance is fully documented in the investigation on the Uses of Social Sciences, conducted by Harold Orlans for the US House Sub-committee on Research led by Henry S. Reuss.

[2] The point has been stressed by Bacon for science in general, in *Valerius Terminus*.

[3] I say 'modal' because it seems to me that there is no 'average' way of life, there is a most frequent way that is 'modal'.

[4] Thus for instance, if I may be so anecdotal, my book *On Power* (1948) arose from a historical review of the increase in the social dimension of war.

[5] It seems unnecessary here to stress that anti-pollution policies shall imply some mix of *ex ante* measures (prescribed decrease of emission) implying increased producer costs, and of *ex post* measures (cleaning up) implying government expenditures.

References

BACON, FRANCIS, *Valerius Terminus*.

BUCHANAN, C., *Traffic in Towns*. HMSO, London, 1963.

DE JOUVENEL, B., *On Power*. (Translation) Hutchinson, London, 1948.

— *L'Art de la conjecture*. Éditions du Rocher, Paris, 1964.

MARX, K., and ENGELS, F., *Manifesto of the Communist Party*. London, 1848.

MONTESQUIEU, C. L., *The Spirit of the Laws*. Paris, 1748.

PLINY, *Natural History*. Book 2, Chapters CV and CVI.

POLANYI, M., *Personal Knowledge: Towards a Post-critical Philosophy*, Routledge and Kegan Paul, London, 1958.

PRICE, D. K., *The Scientific Estate*. Harvard University Press, Cambridge, Mass., 1965.

QUÉTELET, A., *Sur l'homme et le développement de ses facultés, ou essai de physique sociale*. 2 Vols, Paris, 1835.

SPROUT, H. M., *The Ecological Perspective in Human Affairs, with Special Reference to International Politics*. Princeton University Press, Princeton, N.J., 1965.

Interchapter

Because of the enormous growth of science, in both resources and prestige, that has occurred, particularly over the last quarter of a century, together with the minor and insecure standing that has been awarded to the social sciences, many social scientists see the growth of their disciplines coming about by following in the footsteps of the natural sciences.

Differences in the kinds of knowledge sought and the ways of thinking between the natural sciences and the social sciences make the model of the natural sciences inappropriate to the social sciences. However, in so far as the growth in the natural sciences and their technologies has come about because of a belief in their ability to supply some of the needs and wants of man, then this may point to a role that the social sciences should play.

De Jouvenel emphasized this point by quoting again from Bacon 'to make distribution of sciences, arts, inventions, works and their portions according to the use and tribute which they yield and render to the conditions of man's life'.

It is becoming more apparent that many of the needs and wants of man will be supplied by applying the social rather than the natural sciences, and hence more and more often the social sciences are being called upon to help in problem-solving. But this is not to say that the social sciences have the capacity to accept this role. The first task of social scientists is to prove to policy-makers and to society at large that they have the capacity for problem-solving; their second task is to develop this capacity.

The use of social science in problem-solving has been called applied social science. Professor de Jouvenel found the implications behind this term rather worrying. It implies that social scientists have developed a theoretical framework for explaining all social phenomena, and that this can then be applied to each and every individual problem. This is obviously far from the truth, and raises the issue of whether the social scientists should concentrate on what de Jouvenel calls 'what-to-do problems'. He himself strongly favoured the latter approach, and used one economist's description of Keynes's theory to illustrate this – how intellectually satisfying, how aesthetically pleasing, is the structure of the Grand Theory, but how inadequate in taking notice of unemployment and attacking it as a problem.

Trist agreed that we have insufficient theoretical background to solve problems internally from our models because we must go 'into the field' to determine our problems. By allowing oneself to respond to one's society and becoming engaged with whatever opportunities presented themselves, we advance fundamental social science. Any conclusions, concepts, models we may then draw from our research will be closely linked to 'reality'. Yet these will not be global generalizations, or grand theories but 'grounded' concepts. Cherns's thesis that 'the more usable the less generalizable' (see Chapter 2) points to the need for theories grounded in action and generalizable to classes of action.

If social scientists choose to be involved with concrete problems, they become implicated with power agencies, who will commission the research and will try to determine which areas are appropriate for social science research, and which are not. How, then, can the social scientist maintain what he considers to be his right – his freedom of inquiry? How can social scientists reconcile their own values and political opinions to the idea of the disinterested researcher, while carrying out problem-oriented social research?

Brim emphasized this as a very serious problem facing the social science community in America – a problem glossed over in the several recent reports from government bodies involved in social science research. Both Rokkan and Jolles added that this is by no means a uniquely American problem, but one of the burning issues facing the social science community everywhere. We are being challenged by policy-makers and sponsors of research, but even more strongly by our younger colleagues, to show how our disciplines are relevant to the alleviation of our many discontents. But if the ideals of value-free research, of disinterestedness, are anachronistic, what right have we to freedom of inquiry and autonomy in our research?

In presenting his paper, Professor de Jouvenel raised the point, which was again taken up in discussion, of the role of the social scientist as predictor. De Jouvenel was interested both in research on the future (futurology) and in the use of statistics. Statistics can only be used to describe past or present events, and can describe phenomena only when they have been recognized; statistics cannot therefore be used to predict new or changing phenomena in society. Many people have been led to ask how it is, with all our study of society, that we failed to foresee the 'Events of May' in France in 1968, or why, when most political behaviour in Northern Ireland has a historical explanation, the civil disturbances of 1969 should take us by surprise.

Does the answer lie in the intellectual conservatism that characterizes much of today's social science? This theme, the need for 'imagination stretching', was raised again in the session on social indicators.

2 Social sciences and policy

Albert Cherns

The first three chapters of this book examine social science as a policy area. How are the social sciences used in policy-making; at what stages of the policy process are social science inputs likely to be demanded? The study of policy-making, particularly at the level of national governments, has been neglected in contemporary political science, although through recent developments in areas such as policy analysis and through greater emphasis on the importance of policy contents, the topic is taking on a more sharply defined focus. Hence, there exists a need to understand the processes by which policies are made and, in particular, to determine how such processes are influenced by the content of the issue being considered, by the values and perspectives of the actors involved in the process, by the structures in which the actors are located, and by the environments encompassing these structures.

In his paper, Albert Cherns draws attention to the need to adopt an analytical framework when examining the relationship between social science knowledge and policy. It is too easy and too facile, he argues, to approach the problem from the simplistic viewpoint of the application of research. Rather, the sociology of knowledge must be used to provide an analytical base and hence to develop an accurate understanding of the policy-making process, and of the relationships between knowledge users and knowledge producers. Cherns then discusses possible points of entry for social science into political systems and possible uses of social science inputs, particularly in clarifying policy options. The variety of relationships that may exist between social scientist and policy-maker is also examined, as are the different impacts of differing categories of research.

Formerly Scientific Secretary of the UK Social Science Research Council, Albert Cherns is currently Professor of Social Sciences at the University of Loughborough, UK, where he is also Director of the Centre for the Utilization of Social Science Research. His major research interests and recent publications are in the areas of the organization, utilization, and diffusion of social science research.

INTRODUCTION AND SUMMARY

In this paper I try to show that the social sciences have contributed to policy by:

(i) providing the policy-maker with theories, good or bad, about man and about society which underpin his decisions;
(ii) providing data; and
(iii) occasionally devising technical solutions to problems.

Attempts to determine the relationship of social science knowledge to policy have proved a barren task, partly because this has been seen in terms of the application of research rather than the sociology of knowledge. Thus the prospectus under which social research has been offered is a false one.

Unrecognized by both social scientists and policy-makers, ideological assumptions underlie not only the identification of research problems but also the choice of research methodology, and have influenced policy.

The relationships between policy-makers and researchers are critical to the successful identification of problems for research and the utility of the outcome of the research. Successful use of the social sciences involves accurate knowlege of the policy-making process. Only recently has this been studied from the point of view of the social scientist. A fuller understanding aids both in the identification of problems accessible to research and in identification of the processes whereby research can actually aid policy.

WHERE POLICY IS PERMEABLE

The policy-maker, however elevated, however humble, operates on the basis of values, theories, and facts.

It is on the basis of values that the policy-maker prefers one goal to another, thus determining his choice of ends. On the basis of other values which he holds the policy-maker prefers one route to his goal to another, thus determining his choice of means. But the belief that the means he adopts is likely to lead to the end he seeks is based on his theories about the nature of the system he is controlling, or which he is operating. In the case of social systems, or indeed any system in which human beings are involved, his theories must include theories about the nature of man.

On the basis of his theories about cause and effect in the system, the policy-maker has views about facts. He has views as to what facts are relevant and should be taken into account in coming to a decision and views about the reliability of his sources of information.

Thus his values and theories will not only determine the policy-maker's choice of ends and choice of means, but also the knowledge he has about the present state of his system, the further information he will seek, and his evaluation of it when required. They will also, in particular, determine the significance he will attach to social science as a source of relevant knowledge.

What we have described so far has the makings of a perfectly closed system. However, ends are sought, means are selected, actions taken as a result of which the state of the system is changed. This new state must then be compared with the desired state. Any discrepancy is likely to lead to a re-evaluation. The least painful re-evaluation to make is of the facts. If a re-reading of these cannot explain the discrepancy the policy-maker may re-examine his theories.

If, then, we wish to introduce new or different ideas or theories our most hopeful point of entry is at the stage of re-evaluation following the appearance of wide discrepancies between aim and achievement.

STRATEGY OF THE GAPS

The strategy of pointing to the discrepancy between aim and achievement has not escaped the social scientist. In promoting this claim to a place in the political sun social scientists have, by and large, sought to adopt two strategies of which this is one. The other has been to point to the successful uses of social science in policy-making. The search for plausible examples of such successes has usually been abandoned in sorrow. The evidence as far as it exists is in terms of instrumental contributions by social scientists, particularly psychologists, to immediate problems such as how to persuade American housewives to change their families' food habits in wartime.

My own experience is relevant here. In 1959 I first became involved in the problems of the distribution of public money to social science research as Secretary of the Human Sciences Committee of the Department of Scientific and Industrial Research. The very small annual sum of money that that committee was allowed to disburse was to be devoted to 'research in the human sciences related to the needs of industry'. The committee soon felt the need for more money to support a reasonable proportion of the studies seeking its support. I was therefore instructed to prepare an impassioned plea for more money from the Council for Scientific and Industrial Research. The reply to my plea was: 'First show us what we and our predecessors [the joint DSIR/MRC Committees which had spent mainly American counterpart aid funds] have bought with the money so far spent.' It was no use my pointing out that this was the kind of question the Council forbore to ask of its committees supporting the natural sciences. Nor was it of much avail to point to the long time-cycle of utilization (Stansfield, 1967). The Council could afford to demonstrate its hard-headedness on so weak a suppliant. All I could do was to go back to the studies supported by the joint committees, many of which had after all been explicitly aimed at industrial applications, and to follow their progress into utilization, if any. I found scarcely one clear case of deliberate application of a specific finding or recommendation. But I could produce evidence from people in industry that they had been influenced by research, that they had learned from it, and that they thought it a good thing for more research to be undertaken – provided the government paid for it. We got our money.

When the Heyworth Committee was later set up to review the needs of the social sciences, it quickly abandoned the search for specific histories of utilization. It is easy to show that questions of the kind: 'What *specific* use has been made of research in the social sciences?' are misconceived. As I show below, research can only have specific use if it is conceived as taking a narrow view of the problem it is tackling and has a strategy for its use designed into its methodology. Research of this kind turns out to have low generalizability which does not necessarily mean, but often does, that it is also trivial.

Much of the trouble lies in our notions about the application of research. We tend to have sophisticated ideas about it when we discuss it in terms of 'sociology of knowledge', but to revert to simplistic models when we are arguing about 'application' and 'applied research'. I have argued elsewhere (Cherns, 1968) that we take over a model derived from a false reading of the translation of research in the natural sciences into technological developments. Thus we continually hear talk on the one hand of the many 'problems' that could be 'solved' by the sponsorship of appropriate social science research and, on the other hand, of the need for protected support for the social sciences to enable them to grow to adulthood when they will be able to solve problems.

However, the search for 'uses' continues: I know of four attempts to trace out the uses made by the US Federal Government and its agencies in social science – the study of Gene Lyons (1969) and the reports by the National Science Foundation (1969), by the National Academy of Sciences (1968), and by the Senate sub-committee on Government Operations (1967). These last four volumes, *Use of Social Research in Federal and Domestic Programs*, are of especial interest mainly because they disclose an extraordinary state of affairs. Whatever else social scientists have to their credit or discredit, they do not seem to have been backward in obtaining funds for research related to the missions of agencies of government. In 1968 Federal expenditure on research in the social sciences, including psychology, amounted to an estimated $333 million. Yet in response to congressional inquiry, agencies could not describe the use that had been made of previous research. This should not really be surprising. No system had been set up for evaluating the research that has been done, nor are criteria for utilization built in to the designs of research projects and programmes. Under these conditions it is hard to see what answers could be expected to questions about utilization. Yet committees of social scientists are set up to inquire into the adequacy of existing research and predictably each recommends more research and more use of research. Committees' reports do not tell you about the disappointments encountered in the search. For this you must turn to the report of the Senate sub-committee or to *The Uses of Sociology* (Lazarsfeld *et al.*, 1968):

> One can understand with hindsight, but it came as a surprise, to realise how difficult it is to find out how and where sociology is being used. The Loomises . . . wrote to several hundred research sociologists about the uses of sociology; only those who were actively connected with some administrative enterprise could give concrete examples . . . a questionnaire was sent to the members of the A.S.A. Section on Medical Sociology; the majority of the respondents had only vague ideas of what happened to their own work. Clients seemed to be more likely to know of uses than the sociologists themselves. But not only are clients difficult to sample; they are often corporations, in which the officers who may have acted on the basis of a report are not easily traced.

Thus the preferred strategy is to point to problems that social science knowledge would help to solve or to ameliorate. Here committees and individual lobbyists have no difficulty at all. The easiest part of the Heyworth Report (1965) to write was no doubt the section outlining the *potential* uses of social science research.

These are usually formulated in terms of *information* that would be of value to policy-makers; very seldom do we find reference to the ways in which better theories and better techniques could help policy-makers. While it is no doubt true that better information makes for better decisions, it is equally true that however good or complete the information available, it will be evaluated in terms of the policy-maker's theories and values, and that mistaken theories and inappropriate values figure as largely in bad decisions as does inadequate information. Fortunately social science is at least as relevant to the choice of theory and value as to the provision of data.

The social scientist who wishes his research to be used cannot just assume that the truths he reveals will find their own way into application. He has an input he wishes to make to an action system of some kind. This action system includes decisions and people who make decisions. Different systems and different components of the same system can use different kinds of input. Without understanding and analysis of the system our social scientist can only fire his arrows into the air. They will, of course, come to earth, he knows not where. Likewise, without an adequate scanning mechanism the decision-maker cannot locate the appropriate sources of input for his needs; he can only expose himself to any arrows that happen to be in the air.

But all this is to assume that the social scientist wants his 'findings' to be used. Some do. Many more want to be published and preferably read, or, more to the point, cited. Many of the most prestigious social scientists operate in a system whose reward structure is oblivious to 'uses', but very permeable to lists of publications and citations by other scholars.

The social scientist, then, who wants to influence policy can look to several points in the policy process where social science knowledge can be influential. We can consider first the process of selecting options, secondly that of realizing the option selected.

POINTS OF ENTRY

(*a*) *Choice of Options*

(*i*) *System Characteristics* Social scientists through theory and analysis can *describe* the system[1] in which the policy-maker is operating, but their choice of descriptive terms is itself value laden and influenced by their views as to what the 'system' is. For example, some sociologists have described and analysed the system of education in England as a mechanism for distributing social rewards and opportunities and thus either advancing or retarding certain aspects of social change. Others may see our system of education as a mechanism for distributing limited resources to maximize more or less traditional types of learning and knowledge. The trouble is that a 'system of education' is both these and more besides. Thus the task, even if we wished to undertake it, of completely describing and analysing the 'system' is probably impossible. However, we can obtain the policy-maker's view of the goals of the system, though even these are likely to be changed or at least modified by our attempt to elucidate them. If the policy-maker understands and accepts this description, he will then be in a better position to assess both the options that are available to him and the likely outcomes of his choice.

(*ii*) *Theories about the Nature of Man* The system to which we have referred in (*i*) is composed very largely of the interactions of people with people, and with machines and other inanimate objects. The possible states that the system can have depend on the nature of the elements of which it is composed and of their interactions. Our estimate of the attainability of any particular state depends on our theories about the nature of the elements. For example, we may conclude that a state of peace between social groups is impossible because of the aggressive nature of man. By influencing the policy-maker's view of the nature of man, social science will affect his assessment of the goals he can hope to achieve, and of their attainability.

Thus by increasing the policy-maker's knowledge and understanding of the system in which he is operating and the characteristics and potentialities of its human components, social science knowledge can clarify and increase the options available to him.

(b) Realizing Options

In choosing the means to attain his ends, the policy-maker needs:

(i) accurate knowledge about the present state of the system;
(ii) the economic, social, and political costs of the possible means he can employ;
(iii) the anticipated consequences of the means he is considering; including
(iv) the possible side-effects of each means, both favourable (fall-out) and unfavourable (backfirings).

Here the contributions of the social sciences are technical rather than analytic. To contribute to (i) the social sciences have developed techniques of measurement – statistical sampling, questionnaire measures of attitudes, and so forth. The technique of cost-benefit analysis provides the knowledge of (ii). Though continually advancing in subtlety cost-benefit analysis has so far carried with it a concealed inference on both values and the theory of the nature of man. By providing a single economic dimension on to which non-economic factors can be projected, cost-benefit analysis has tended to sustain an economic value system by extending its capacity to cope with criticism from social value systems. By linking all social benefits to the cash nexus it has reinforced the theory of economic man, albeit at the cost of widening somewhat the referent of the adjective 'economic'. While we cannot go further into or attempt to do justice to methods of cost-benefit analysis and their influence, their importance in this context is greatest for (iii), the anticipated consequences of means. It enables the policy-maker to anticipate certain consequences but does not alert him to others.

Cost-benefit analysis here offers a good example of the difficulties inherent in almost any attempt to analyse a total system. If it is to be intellectually coherent it must offer a scheme of analysis which brings into measurable relationship with one another all the ramifications of policy decisions. But in any large system we need to break the problem down into examinable entities. These entities are subsystems. Even if we can provide solutions which optimize the operations of all the subsystems, these solutions will not necessarily add up to an optimum solution for the operation of the total system. Perhaps the most promising use of cost-benefit analysis is to identify the options that are available. When used properly it compares the costs and benefits of one solution with the costs and benefits of alternatives. Among the alternatives brought forward for this technical comparison may be some that have been overlooked or ruled out of court on mistaken or irrelevant grounds (Wildavsky, 1966).

As far as (iv) is concerned careful historical analysis of the unanticipated consequences of previous decisions provides the only useful technique to date.

Thus the social sciences have, to some extent, provided the policy-maker with *techniques for realizing options* through aiding him in his selection of means.

After selecting his options and the means whereby they will be achieved the policy-maker may now seek assistance in publicizing his intentions and obtaining a favourable public response. Here again the social sciences can provide technical solutions. A single person may be responsible for all the choices – of goal, of means, and of public relations. In an organization, however, these choices are likely to be made at different and descending levels. Indeed only the first may be truly regarded as policy. To the top level, choice of goal is policy, choice of means is execution of policy. At the next level the choice of means may be a policy decision, execution to take place at a lower level still. However, it is likely that advice on choice of goal will be sought, if at all, by the top echelon; advice on means will be sought at a lower level; and advice on selling a decision at yet another level. Not only will such advice be sought by different echelons, it is likely to be sought from different sources. As we shall see later, this has large implications for the strategy of social science in engaging with organizations.

SOCIAL SCIENCES AND THE MECHANISMS FOR ARTICULATING PUBLIC POLICY

We have so far discussed the ways in which social science can aid the policy-makers. We now turn to examine the ways in which the social sciences relate to existing policy-making processes, and the extent to which existing mechanisms for articulating public policy rely on, or are underpinned by, contributions from the social sciences.

As we shall see, these contributions are of two kinds: mechanisms for obtaining data relevant to the publics concerned; and assumptions derived often from social science methods used to obtain the data.

Inputs to the policy-making process include statistics and survey data as well as the publications of social scientists. These inputs are both direct and indirect. Governments and other policy-making bodies utilize and set great store upon data of a quantitative nature provided by censuses of population, production, and so forth and by surveys of various kinds – in Britain the government has ready recourse to findings from its own Social Survey. Political parties in or out of office are, of course, influenced in their policy-making by results of polls, some commissioned specially. Social science methods of obtaining quantitative representations of social benefits are now increasingly used in cost-benefit analysis studies preceding decisions on public investment. Statistical data of every kind are sought eagerly by policy-making bodies and skilled interpretation of the data and trends from these statistics are both required and relied upon.

The first point I wish to make is that the social sciences have played the predominant part in the origin of the statistics and of methods of obtaining, evaluating, and presenting them and treating them to yield economic and social indicators of various kinds. Any consideration of the use of the social sciences in policy-making must take these facts into account.

The second point is that statistics are by no means value free, nor necessarily are the mathematical methods used in extracting the information for use. They rest on theories and even on ideologies. To begin with, statistics have, until very recently at any rate, been virtually confined to what could be measured or counted. (Often what can be counted or measured has been identified with the logical and rational; what could not be counted or measured was irrational or metaphysical.) Thus there has been a tendency to undervalue the immeasurable or uncountable. Second, some procedures have embodied an unstated and probably unrealized ideological assumption. The counting of heads implies the equivalence of heads, or at least the propriety of treating the individual as the unit. It is one thing to sample the opinions of all adults in a community; another to sample the opinions of heads of families, villages, tribes, or whatnot. Our democratic, one-person/one-vote, ideology infects the choice of data and method of acquiring it. When we choose the individual as our unit we imply both that the matter is one which appropriately refers to individuals as units and that individuals are equal units for the purpose. I am not attacking democracy; I am pointing out that its ideology is implicit in many of our 'objective' methods and data.

Furthermore, our methods of obtaining data are overwhelmingly verbal. Questionnaires, interviews, censuses are conducted through the use of verbal symbols; some behaviour is much more accessible to verbal report than others; what is less accessible is largely ignored. We prefer 'hard' methods to those more difficult to assess and replicate (La Piere, 1934). We prefer questionnaire data to participant observation; surveys have prospered, 'mass observation' has become unfashionable. All this is perfectly proper provided we know what we are doing. But we don't know, or we forget.

Some measures, indicators, are available which do not rely on verbal report. So far they have been little used. Some are reported in *Unobtrusive Measures*. These, it is true, still rely on some quantitative measures or observations (Webb *et al.*, 1966).

Proposals current in the United States since the late 1920s for the development of social indicators to set alongside the more prominent economic indicators are, if adopted, likely to have the effects of drawing attention to non-economic issues, but still to the more easily measurable aspects of social issues.

POLICY-MAKING AND DECISION-MAKING

Before I go on to discuss the relationship between policy-maker and researcher – which I consider to be a crucial issue – I need to make a distinction between policy-making and decision-making. This distinction is not always very clearly made. Sometimes policy is treated as identical with administrative action. (See R. K. Merton's discussion (1949) of 'the world of practical decision'.) Potentially we weaken the argument for the role of the social sciences if we let it be thought that we are claiming their relevance to all decision-making. A close reading of Merton's article and, in particular, of his taxonomy of research objectives makes it clear that he is thinking of policy objectives, not of decision-making *per se*. He classifies research problems into:

> Diagnostic (e.g. providing information on whether the situation has changed); Prognostic (e.g. forecasting future needs); Differential prognosis (e.g. selecting options); Evaluative (e.g. comparing performance with aim); together with general background data such as: 'Educative' research (e.g. setting out the true facts for the public) and

Strategic fact-finding (e.g. systematic purposive assembling of descriptive data) (Merton, 1949).

This classification, though logically incomplete, can make sense as policy research only if all policy is taken to have a programmatic referent. However, policy may not be programmatic though it is distinguished from decision-making by being iterative. Rose (1969) points out that:

> Policy-making involves a long series of more or less related activities rather than a single, discrete decision . . . It thus covers far more than the term decision-making. The study of decision-making usually involves analysing the intentions of policy-makers up to and including the point at which binding . . . action is taken . . . Outcomes may be affected less by conscious decision to act than by conscious or unconscious preferences for inaction . . . The sense of continuous activity and adjustment involved in policy-making is best conveyed by describing it as a process, rather than a single once-for-all act.

Unfortunately, Snyder and Paige (1958) define decision-making as:

> . . . a sequence of activities which results in selection of one course of action intended to bring about the particular future state of affairs envisaged by the decision-makers.

This is almost identical with our chosen definition of policy-making. We do need definitions, though they need not be too precise. We shall therefore read policy for decision in Snyder and Paige's description, stressing again the continuity involved in policy. If policy-making then is not a once-for-all affair, can the effective contribution of social science be a once-for-all affair? Rather I would maintain that the sequential nature of decision-making in policy offers a number of points where social science research can make an input. Furthermore it allows for a more developed relationship between researcher and policy-maker.

RELATIONSHIP BETWEEN POLICY-MAKER AND SOCIAL SCIENTIST

Whether the role of the social scientist is described as one of adviser or consultant, researcher or even critic, his relationship with the policy-maker is essentially one of provider of knowledge. This knowledge may, as we have indicated, take different forms: it may be an analytical framework; new facts or new relationships between previously known facts. The knowledge to be usable must have validity for the client.

Niehoff (1966) discusses the ways in which knowledge must be adapted to pass effectively from one culture system to another. He refers to the 'sociocultural component, which means simply that technical knowhow and economic patterns are embedded in cultural systems, elaborate patterns of customs and beliefs, which can either act as sanctions or barriers to technical or economic change'. It seems that it is legitimate to spell this out with a wealth of examples for American would-be change agents going overseas; it is more presumptuous to point to the differences between administrative and academic cultures or among different administrative cultures as obstacles to acceptance of the validity of social science knowledge. Nevertheless, we are not entitled to assume that all administrative organizations in our society are equally ready to accept the legitimacy of ideas. Hauser (1967) has made the point that in a complex society we have 'almost every stage of social evolution simultaneously present'. Thus different politicians in the United States 'talk past one another. They can't even understand the frames of reference with which they are involved.' This may be putting it strongly, but even an overstatement is a valuable corrective to the bland assumption that what is seen as valid knowledge in one frame of reference will necessarily be similarly accepted in another.

Warren Bennis (1961) has sketched what is required for knowledge generated by the social sciences to be 'valid'. His 'desiderata' include taking into consideration 'the behaviour of persons operating within their specific institutional environment', accepting that groups and organizations are 'as amenable to empirical and analytical treatment as the individual', and, above all, including 'variables the practitioner can understand, manipulate and evaluate'. But even the most heroic efforts to generate 'valid' knowledge will fail if the 'practitioner', as Bennis calls him (or, as he sometimes refers to him generically, the 'client system'), or, in our terms, the policy-maker, fails to generate the corresponding capacity to assimilate the knowledge provided.

Thus these are desiderata for a social science that can, in my belief, generate valid knowledge only if the 'client system' generates the corresponding capacity to assimilate the knowledge provided. Above all, it must have, or must develop, channels for diffusion of the 'valid' knowledge. Lazarsfeld *et al.* (1968) describe this problem:

> Whatever study has been made, whatever fund of available knowledge has been drawn upon, then comes the moment when one has to make the *leap from knowledge* to decision.

First, of course, following Bennis, we can say that the knowledge has not only to be 'available', but also 'valid'. But the concern of the social scientist cannot end at the point where he has made valid knowledge available to the policy-maker. He must also, if he is concerned with the usability of, as well as the validity of, this knowledge, be concerned with the policy-maker's capability of adopting the conceptual base into which the knowledge can be absorbed so as to make the leap from a secure platform. This means among other things that the policy-maker and social scientist must have similar conceptions of the relationship of science to policy. Horowitz (1967) points out that social scientists are anxious to study the policy process so as to add to scientific knowledge, as well as providing 'intelligence' for government, whereas the policy-makers in government are more interested in social engineering than in social science. Horowitz makes two further important points: first, that while policy places a premium on involvement and influence, science places a premium on investigation and ideas. The issue is not so much what is studied or even the way an inquiry is conducted but the auspices and purposes of a study. Second, that what one witnesses in the social sciences is the break-up of the functionalist ideology with its value-free orientation. This last point we must take up again in consideration of the ethical problems of the relationship of the social sciences to policy. It is important here because it shows that Bennis's valid knowledge is knowledge acquired from a particular standpoint and cannot in any way be regarded as value-free scientific knowledge. However this may reflect on the scientific status of the knowledge, it certainly implies that the valid knowledge provided by the social scientist is based on a shared system of values between the social scientist and the policy-maker.

Churchman and Emery (1966) argue the consequences of this very cogently. They discuss the relationship between the organization to which the researcher belongs and the organization which he is studying. They consider three ideal types of this relationship.

> One approach . . . is to regard the researcher as a member of an organization completely independent of the organization being observed.

In this type of relationship the researcher's reference group is the research community with its values of scientific objectivity and disinterestedness and purity. His goals are publication, a scientifically sound piece of work, and the recognition of the scientific community. As a member of an entirely different kind of organization from that which he is studying he may not find it possible to identify the organization's problems in terms which meet its real needs. Nor can the research organization learn how to make its output more valuable to the organization it studies.

> A second approach to the study of organizations is to regard the researcher as both a member of an independent research community

> and a member *pro tem* of another organization that includes the one being observed (Churchman and Emery, 1966).

Here the researcher is faced with insoluble dilemmas. He cannot resolve conflicts in the goals of the two organizations. He has to restrict his involvement in the organization under study and therefore shies away from problems of central importance. Further he has conflicting claims on his time. Should he end the research when the research organization is satisfied or go on until the observed organization accepts and understands his contribution?

> A third approach to the study of organizations is to regard the researcher as a member *pro tem* of a third organization sufficiently greater than the organization under study to encompass the conflicting interests and yet sufficiently close to it to permit its values to be related to the concrete issues of conflict (Churchman and Emery, 1966).

In this view we escape the problem of the social scientist's acquiring the values of the policy-maker by requiring that both share values sanctioned by a higher-level organization of which both are members. At the level of their interaction the policy-maker has acquired a capability of using knowledge whose validity is not determined by its relevance to his view as an administrator or the aim and functioning of his organization. Policy-maker and researcher are then able to engage in the mutual learning approach, which is the most effective way in which knowledge generated by social science research can be brought into the action frame of reference of the policy-maker. The basis for this mutual learning must however be continually shifting.

The question then arises: how much shift in the basis of the 'shared agreements' can take place without overstraining the tension between the policy-maker and the researcher? At what point do roles undergo so much change that the basis of negotiation has been changed, requiring new roles? And if new roles are required, can they be assumed without a change of cast?

G. N. Jones (1969) has introduced the definition of three roles involved in the processes of change in policy in organizations. These roles are 'change agent', 'change catalyst', and 'pacemaker'.

The 'change agent' is a 'helpful professional'. Like the 'client system' he possesses his own unique set of values, norms, and behavioural patterns. The change catalyst examines widespread influence at small cost to himself. He may at one stage facilitate the interaction of change agent and client system and is at all times free to move between them. The pacemaker, which may be an individual, group, or organization, has as its primary function the maintenance of the change process 'by the proper and the systematic changes of stimuli'.

At different stages during the consideration and adoption of policy changes using knowledge generated by social science research, the three functions of agent, catalyst, and pacemaker become crucial and remain of importance for different durations. All three functions can be fulfilled by social scientists or at any rate by people with some training in the social sciences. They cannot be filled by the same social scientist as they involve different sets of relationship with the policy-maker. Difficulties arise in practice because as the basis of the 'shared agreement' shifts, demands are made first on one then on another of these roles. Simple models relating one researcher to one policy-maker ignore the variety and complexities of these relationships and ignore, too, the fact that both policy-maker and researcher must operate within organizational contexts.

A TYPOLOGY OF RESEARCH

Not only are we obliged to consider different relationships between policy-maker and researcher at different stages of the policy process, we also need to consider the different relationships appropriate to different kinds of research.

Elsewhere (Cherns, 1969) I have tried to show that different types of research have associated with them different channels of diffusion. I have described these as:

(i) *Pure Basic Research*, arising out of the perceived needs of the discipline, oriented towards resolving or elucidating or exemplifying a theoretical problem. The diffusion channel typically associated with this type of research is the academic publication. Because it is an 'open' channel, random or fortunately directed scanning by policy-makers *may* pick up its output. More frequently it has to pass first through other channels before entering those associated with action.

(ii) *Basic Objective Research*, oriented towards a problem that arises in some field of application, but not aimed at prescribing a particular solution. The typical diffusion channel is the same as (i) but much more frequently the research is communicated to 'professional' as distinct from 'academic' journals and is fed through specialist teaching (e.g. of managers) into action channels.

(iii) *Operational Research*, aimed at tackling an ongoing problem within an organizational framework, but not including experimental action.

The typical diffusion channel is feedback straight to the administrators of the organization.

(iv) *Action Research*, involving introducing and observing planned change. Here the feedback link is similar to that in (iii) but is continuous during the period of the research.

Of these only (iii) and (iv) have diffusion channels associated with them which involve the completion of a feedback link into action. Typically operational research relies on diffusion into the policy channels, at the completion of the study, to generate the pressure for the recommended action. The design of action research builds in action on recommendations by a series of feedback loops linked to one another by the start and end of each increment of planned experimental change. The paradox here is that as the generality of action research and operational research is low compared to that of basic research, the more generality and hence potential utility the research possesses, the weaker the system by which it may enter action-decision channels.

One may note in this analysis no mention of 'applied' research. Types (ii), (iii), and (iv) are all in a sense applied research. The trouble with the term 'applied' is that it begs the question. 'Applied' refers to the intention not the outcome of the research. And unless it is designed as operational or action research, the 'applied' research is conducted without reference to the subsequent diffusion of results into action channels. The literature bristles with examples of research undertaken with an applied objective which have with outstanding luck illuminated a theoretical problem, with ordinary luck contributed to the growing stock of reportable or teachable case studies. The luckless remainder have reached the final resting-place of most research – the policy-maker's pigeon-hole. (A new outcome has become possible, a case study in the pack of illustrations of the difficulties of obtaining utilization of applied research.) Few cases of documented utilization are reported. But as no provision was made for building utilization into the design of the research we should not be surprised. Yet apparently Lazarsfeld, Sewell, and Wilensky (1968) were.

Different types of research institutions are linked to different diffusion channels. For example, universities are linked with the channels of academic publication; independent research institutions and business schools are more likely to use 'professional' channels; in-house research units are more likely to undertake operational or action research.

The time characteristics of the policy-administrative process set many specific problems for research. It is not only a question of the policy-maker's need for quick results nor his difficulties in attempting to predict what will be his future needs for research. Different kinds of information are needed at different phases of the policy process. Analytic studies classifying and possibly increasing options are required at the stage when options are being generated and considered. Technical studies are needed at the stage of realizing options. Manipulative 'research' may be called for (and in some instances some social scientists would not regard this as totally improper) at the stage of obtaining acceptance of the favoured option. For example, researchers may be asked to find out how a particular policy can be 'sold'. Or they may be asked to undertake research aimed to 'show the need for XYZ'. A third example of manipulative research may be to make findings selectively available. For an instance of this see Rainwater and Yancey (1967). And the time characteristics of the phases of the policy-making process and of the associated researches can be expected to match only in action research (which cannot otherwise be undertaken).

Following this analysis it would seem that the linkage between policy-making and social science can be improved by changes in the mutual perceptions of policy-maker and social scientist, and their joint understanding of the potential relevance of research and the problems of diffusion of its results into channels of action and policy-making. A greater planned range of research institutions with special competences in one or other kind of research would doubtless help too. But we can get just so far with tailoring research to assist in the formulation and realization of policy. At least as much advantage could come from using the resources of social science to *improve the policy-making process.*

SOCIAL SCIENCE AND THE POLICY-MAKING PROCESS

The style and time-scale of policy-making, and the quantity of research information that must be processed, will vary with other significant parameters, including the reactiveness of the environment or, in Emery's (1968) terms, its 'turbulence'. Policy-makers in large systems, ranging from corporations and universities to governments, are operating more and more in turbulent fields of this kind. Policies of an incremental kind are likely to be futile in non-linear systems. The policy-maker is, therefore, faced with situations in which not only is he unable to predict the effects of different possible decisions; he may be unable to relate consequences to actions. His problem is worse confounded if the system's time characteristics are such that it responds sluggishly to his actions. Successive Chancellors of the Exchequer in Britain may recognize this situation! Can the social sciences help to devise improved schemata for policy-making in this type of situation? Emery (1968) points to 'systems management' as a possible schema. It involves: selecting and re-selecting goals that appear to be attainable, given the characteristics of the field as well as of the system; applying criteria derived from the goal for comparing means; tighter assessment of results, particularly against interim goals; a 'flexible framework' of information and decision using scientific and other specialized knowledge; control by information, prediction, and persuasion; and better ways of predicting the interactions of simultaneous policy decisions. Turbulent fields cannot be negotiated by traditionally hierarchically structured organizations. Organizational forms able to cope with turbulent fields must develop processes of policy-making that can take into account the social processes that arise through the 'mutual adjustment of the values and interests of the participants'.

This seems a formidable task and we are offered little guidance as to the means by which it can be achieved. Of course, conceptualizing the need is itself a step in the right direction.

However, there is one corresponding advantage. Even though turbulent fields may negate the possibility of comprehensive centralized planning of decision-making, it also means that there need be a less rigid sequence of decision-making (Lindblom, 1958). Points not attended to can be dealt with as they appear because of the successive and serial nature of analysis and policy-making.

What begins to emerge here is a concept, recently adopted in social science, of the 'learning' system – the system that is designed so that it can adjust its behaviour as it encounters reality. We are, of course, witnessing both a backlash against centralized planning and a simultaneous provision of a cloak of respectability for a degree of laissez-faire. But it is clear from what has already been said that centralized planning and control encounters enormous difficulties in turbulent fields. The concept of learning has the right sound of flexibility and growth. It also suggests an organic character to the process and replaces mechanical by biological images. Let us see what this implies. Hirschman and Lindblom (1962) show that a number of lines of thought converge on a model of policy management:

Some policy-making processes and modes of behaviour, ordinarily considered to be irrational and wasteful, are rational and useful.

Some matters need 'wise and salutary neglect'.

One step ought often to be left to lead to another. It is unwise to specify objectives in much detail when the means of attaining them are virtually unknown.

Goals will change through experience with a succession of means-ends and ends-means adjustments.

A rational problem-solver wants what he can get and does not try to get what he wants, except after identifying what he wants by examining what he can get.

The exploration of alternative uses of resources can be overdone.

Decision-makers need to discern and react promptly to newly emerging problems, imbalances, and difficulties. If they are too concerned with eliminating them in advance, by 'integrated planning', they lose the ability to react and to improvise readily and imaginatively.

Since we have limited capacities to solve problems and particularly to foresee the shape of future problems, we may do best the 'hard way' of learning by experience.

These amount to a theory of successive decision-making, relying on the clues that appear in the course of the sequence and concentrating on identification of these clues.

Processes of mutual adjustment of participants are capable of achieving a kind of co-ordination not necessarily centrally envisaged prior to its achievement, or centrally managed.

These points do not amount to a recipe for blind incrementalism, but to a scheme for a re-orientation of the policy-maker to (a) the characteristics of the system he is trying to plan or to control, (b) the characteristics of the behaviour of systems in turbulent fields, and (c) the role of policy-maker. They point to arranging useful learning experiences for the organization; a continual process of reality-testing both of goals and of means. The social sciences can relate to this policy process most effectively in two ways: first, by analysing the nature of the system that the policy-maker is controlling and, secondly, by helping to devise the reality-testing procedures and by monitoring them. While basic research is clearly required for the former, operational and action research techniques will have to be developed on a wide scale to undertake the latter.

Even now when we have outlined roles for the social sciences and for social scientists in assisting in goal-selection as well as means-selecting procedures, we cannot escape totally the problems of values associated with any relationship of science to policy. Granted the impossibility of a value-free social science contribution to policy-making, there is, I think, a role somewhere among the kinds of research mentioned in this paper for all social scientists who count among their values that of assisting in the design and growth of social institutions capable of learning and adapting to the complexities we create by existing.

Note

[1] My use of the word 'system' here is not intended to imply any concomitant to what is described as Systems Theory, beyond the minimum assumption that without some model of the way elements interrelate the policy-maker could not predict the relative outcomes of different actions.

References

BENNIS, W., BENNE, K. D., and CHIN, R., *The Planning of Change*. Holt, Rinehart, and Winston, New York, 1961.

CHERNS, A. B., Uses of the Social Sciences. *Human Relations* **21**, 4, 1968.

— Social Science Research and its Diffusion. *Human Relations* **22**, 3, June, 1969, pp. 210–18.

CHURCHMAN, C. W., and EMERY, F. E., *Operational Research and the Social Sciences*, J. R. Lawrence (ed.). Tavistock Publications, London, 1966.

EMERY, F. E., *Forecasting and the Social Sciences*, M. Young (ed.). Heinemann, London, 1968.

HAUSER, P. M., *Washington Colloquium on Science and Society*, M. Leeds (ed.). Mono Book Corporation, Baltimore, 1967.

Heyworth Report, *Report on Social Studies*. Cmnd 2660, HMSO, London, 1965.

HIRSCHMAN, A. O. and LINDBLOM, C. C., Economic Development, Research and Development, Policy-making: Some Converging Views. *Behavioural Science* **7**, 1962, pp. 212–22.

HOROWITZ, I. L. (ed.), *The Rise and Fall of Project Camelot*. MIT Press, Cambridge, Mass., 1967.

JONES, G. N., *Planned Organisational Change*. Routledge and Kegan Paul, London, 1969.

LA PIERE, R. T., Attitudes versus Actions. *Social Forces*, **13**, 1934, pp. 230–7.

LAZARSFELD, P., SEWELL, W. H., and WILENSKY, H. (eds.), *The Uses of Sociology*. Weidenfeld and Nicholson, London, 1968.

LINDBLOM, C. C., Policy Analysis, *American Economic Review* **48**, 1958, pp. 298–312.

LYONS, GENE M., *The Uneasy Partnership: Social Science and the Federal Government in the Twentieth Century*. Russell Sage Foundation, New York, 1969.

MERTON, R. K., The Role of Applied Social Science in the Formation of Policy, *Philosophy of Science* **16**, No. 3, 1949, pp. 161–81.

National Academy of Sciences/National Research Council, *The Behavioral Sciences and the Federal Government*. Publication 1680, US Government Printing Office, Washington, 1968 (Young Committee).

National Science Foundation, *Knowledge into Action: Improving the Nation's Use of the Social Sciences.* NSB 69–3, US Government Printing Office, Washington, 1969 (Brim Commission).

NIEHOFF, A. H. (ed.), *A Casebook of Social Change.* Aldine Publishing, Chicago, 1966.

RAINWATER, L., and YANCEY, W. L., *The Moynihan Report and the Politics of Controversy.* MIT Press, Cambridge, Mass., 1967.

ROSE, R. (ed.), *Policy-making in Britain.* Free Press, New York; Papermac, London, 1969.

SNYDER, R. C., and PAIGE, G. D., The United States' Decision to Resist Aggression in Korea: The Application of an Analytical Scheme. *Administration Science Quarterly* No. 3, 1958, pp. 341–78.

STANSFIELD, R. G., The Unnoticed Application of the Results of Research. Paper to Section N of the British Association for the Advancement of Science Conference, 1967.

US Government House of Representatives Committee on Government Operations, *Use of Social Research in Federal and Domestic Programs.* US Government Printing Office, Washington, 1967.

WEBB, E., CAMPBELL, P. T., SCHWARTZ, R. D., and SECHREST, L., *Unobtrusive Measures.* Rand McNally, Chicago, 1966.

WILDAVSKY, A., Cost-Benefit Analysis, Systems Analysis and Programme Budgeting. *Public Administration Review* **26**, 1966, pp. 292–310.

Interchapter

Albert Cherns opened this session by highlighting the major points in his paper, which are summarized below. The relationship between the researcher and the policy-maker vitally influences both the successful identification of problems and the utility of the results from research in aiding the solution of those problems. The social scientist must learn to understand the policy-making process, if he wishes for fuller use to be made of social scientists and social science research.

The relationship of the researcher to the policy-maker is essentially one of provider of knowledge: this knowledge may be in the form of data, or techniques for solving problems, or in the form of theories. But it is not enough to generate 'valid' knowledge; consideration must be given to the 'client's' ability to assimilate not only the knowledge provided but also the conceptual base from which it springs. This means that the policy-maker and the social scientist must have similar conceptions of the relationship of science to policy, based on a shared system of values. The strength of this shared system of values that will be necessary will vary with the different forms of relationship between the researcher, the policy-maker, and their organizations.

Very few attempts to show explicitly the use of social science by policy-makers have been successful, and the speaker suggested that this is due to our simplistic models of 'applied research'. Not only must we consider the different forms the relationship between policy-makers and researchers may take, but also what form is appropriate to different stages of the policy process, to different kinds of research activity, and to different research institutions. Perhaps most important of all, we must consider the processes of diffusion of research results into channels of action and policy-making.

Two issues were immediately raised by Dr Crawford. First, who is this person, the policy-maker, that we talk about and, second, what do we mean by the 'use' of social science?

While many of the participants found no difficulty in identifiying policy-makers, there was more general agreement that it could be misleading to use the term policy-maker in such a global fashion. He came in many diverse forms, played many roles, was found in many different institutions, at different levels within those institutions, and acted at different stages in the policy-making process.

But even if we can identify the policy-maker, how can we go about studying the way in which he uses the knowledge provided by the social scientists? Because of the difficulty in pinpointing when a piece of research or knowledge was 'used', Dr Crawford suggested that she would prefer the term 'influence'. The process of influencing the policy-maker will be very different in the case of face-to-face interaction between the policy-maker and the social scientist, compared with the case where knowledge travels on its own, so to speak, from the academic system to the policy-making system.

Agreeing with this, Dr Brim stressed that in trying to increase the influence of social science on policy, we must distinguish between current and long-term strategy. An example of long-term strategy was the increase in the amount of social science teaching and research that was carried out in the US in the professional schools. Many now training to be lawyers, doctors, social workers, or managers, would become the policy-makers of the future; providing them with a basic understanding of the social sciences was one way of advancing, in the long term, the influence of social science on policy-making.

Professor Mendras raised the point, which was discussed at greater length later in the conference, that the social sciences, apart from economics, did not influence the policy-maker, because of differences in the ideology between the two sectors. Economists had been able to convince the policy-makers that they could provide answers to problems, and answers acceptable to the policy-maker – 'they had wheels to turn'. The other social sciences still had to convince the policy-maker that they had something understandable and acceptable to offer to him.

Very few studies had been made of why some research was successful in influencing policy-makers, while others failed. What criteria could be used to assess success or failure? Dr Roberts thought that these criteria may well be different for the social scientists and the policy-maker, while Jeremy Mitchell felt that the difficulty in drawing up criteria for evaluating research in the social sciences lay in the dynamic nature of the problems the social scientist was trying to solve. While the social scientist and the policy-maker may have similar views on the definition of the problem at any one point in time, the nature of the problem may not stay constant during a research programme; hence any criteria established to evaluate the results of the research would rapidly become outmoded.

Several members felt that any attempt to reach a fuller understanding of the impact of social science research on the policy formation process would be aided by the publication of a series of case studies analysing in depth those occasions when a policy-maker asked for the help of social scientists and whether this led to a successful or unsuccessful relationship, with the adoption of social science knowledge into the decision-making process. Professor Jolles, in particular, thought that such a document, written on both a substantive comparative basis and a crossnational basis, would provide invaluable teaching material.

3 Policy-making as a learning process

A work note on social science policy

Einar Thorsrud

Although policy-making is frequently discussed at the level of national government, other areas, both private and public, initiate, implement, and evaluate policies. The function of social science in policy-making at these subsidiary levels is an even more neglected topic for analysis than the relationship between social science and government.

Einar Thorsrud has been closely connected with the use of social science in non-governmental areas and the associated impact over policy-making in these areas. In Chapter 3 he deals in depth with the Industrial Democracy Project in Norway, which he uses to illustrate how policy can emerge step by step through a collaborative relationship between social scientists and users of research. Setting this project in its wider context, he traces its initiation and development, taking account of both internal and external pressures on the accepted definition of the problem and on the emergence of different policy issues at both the institutional and the national levels. Thorsrud's conclusions arising from the analysis of this project are very much of an incrementalist nature in that he sees policy-making as a complex learning process involving many interest groups, hence something that cannot be assessed simplistically, i.e. as a well-ordered systematic process. Further, he stresses the interdependence of social science with other fields – a factor that demands collaborative relationships between social scientists and other parties, and also the need, in any long-term social science programme, to avoid rigid distinctions between theoretical and applied research.

Einar Thorsrud is Research Director of the Work Research Institutes, Oslo, Norway. His major interests are in organizational and industrial sociology and he has played a leading part in the initiation and development of the Norwegian Industrial Democracy Project described in this chapter. Recent publications include: *Form and Content in Industrial Democracy* (with F. E. Emery, 1969); *Towards New Organizational Forms in Enterprise* (with F. E. Emery, 1969).

INTRODUCTION

Shortage of money and the awareness of unsolved problems are usually the main reasons for scientists to ask for a new science policy. In return they are often confronted with this question: 'What *problems* will you solve and how will you *organize* your work?' The question is raised by government and politicians, as well as by industry and others who have the money and the problems. Each expects an answer first to his question. In this way we get a deadlock in policy-making and problem-solving. The gap between the scientific world and society at large broadens and frustration grows on both sides. Science policy committees can usually achieve very little to change this situation.

Real changes in science policy occur

(i) when the size of investments in science and their costs become a threat to other sectors in society,
(ii) when serious problems are not solved by the present allocation of resources.

Overinvestment can hardly be expected soon to cause major changes in social science policy. The case is different for certain sectors of technology and the natural sciences. The gravity of the problems in society that the social sciences could possibly help to solve will perhaps be the major reason for social science policy to emerge. But who can identify those problems and enable the social sciences to approach them in time? This is exactly what a social science policy should help to do. A lack of such policy in the past can be observed if we look at city planning and the educational explosion, the health and welfare services, and the use of human resources in industry. Social scientists are not in a position to claim that they could have done a great deal to solve the pressing problems in present-day society. So far they have in fact done very little. But they have built a body of knowledge and a set of skills that could be tried out in a wide range of community affairs—not only because some problems might be solved, but also for the benefit of scientific development. But can this be done before we have a science policy for the mobilization of larger resources and for guiding the use of such resources? In other words, we are back to the deadlock in policy-making and problem-solving we stated initially.

Social science policy as a collaborative relationship

It is my purpose here to illustrate how policy-making can emerge step by step in a collaborative relationship between social scientists and users of research. Rather than looking at policy-making as a precondition for social science mobilization we will look at it as a learning process.[1] The following major steps can be observed:

(I) initiation of problem identification and preliminary allocation of resources
(II) search for alternative problem-solving activities, building of mutual trust, and sharing of responsibilities
(III) stepwise experimental change
(IV) evaluation and diffusion of results
(V) re-allocation of resources to match environmental changes.

The Industrial Democracy Project

We shall use the Industrial Democracy Project in Norway to illustrate such a learning process. This project started in 1962 with a study of formal representation of employees at board level of companies. Since 1964 a number of field experiments have been carried out to improve the conditions for personal participation in actual work situations. The results have now started to spread in industry and shipping.

I. INITIATION OF PROBLEM IDENTIFICATION AND PRELIMINARY ALLOCATION OF RESOURCES

The research group was impressed by the following characteristics of the situation when the initiation of this research programme took place in 1961–2.

External pressure was felt by industrial and trade union leaders to provide answers to several important problems implicit in the discussion of 'industrial democracy'. The boom in education and the realization of major welfare objectives were followed by new demands in industry. Among them were demands for more meaningful work situations and for a redistribution of social influence. Technological development and international markets had an increasing impact upon the structure of industry on national, regional, and company level. The merging of companies into powerful groups and the growth of international business corporations threatened to limit the choice of organizational patterns according to local values. Human resources rather than raw materials and existing manufacturing technology would form the basis for survival in a world market.

Internal pressure for change was felt inside trade unions as well as in industrial enterprises. In spite of steady economic growth, the low-salary groups and workers in weak industrial regions raised reasonable claims for better pay and for more safety on the job. The radical wing of the labour movement pressed for equalization of power among the major partners in industry, although solutions like nationalization did not attract the majority of workers. Increased alienation in the work situation was felt to have a growing effect upon local initiative in enterprises as well as in unions. Professionally trained specialists and managers were looking for new trends in organizational developments that would enable them to realize their potential capacities.

Institutional co-operation has a long tradition in Scandinavian labour management relations. Although there were obviously different interests at stake in the existing situation, common interests were stronger. Representatives of unions and employers' organizations chose to extend a joint invitation to social scientists to co-operate with them. The need for professional assistance from social scientists seemed clear to both parties, although it was not clear how such assistance could be obtained. The research group welcomed joint responsibility for a project, but could not guarantee that power relationships on national as well as on company level might not change if a research and development programme became effective. The two sponsors each paid 50 per cent of this first phase of the project. Further financing was necessary but was postponed until the first results could be envisaged.

The social scientists had not initiated the project by seeking permission to do a special study, which is usually the starting-point for similar projects. They were quite willing to work with the collaborating parties over some time before they were guaranteed a long-term project or a broader programme. A short-term project would certainly have been of little use to anyone involved, since the problems were obviously not simple. But the social scientists did not expect the other parties to commit themselves to something that could not be well defined at the outset.

The jointly formulated research programme was the result of several meetings of a national committee. Industrial and union leaders brought in their own ideas and those of their organizations. The social scientists brought in the results from previous research and formulated alternative approaches. Labour law and collective bargaining were considered to be an important aspect of industrial democracy in Norway. Improvements could be made but these did not require the assistance of social scientists as much as some other aspects. Several problems in this area were also defined as belonging to the political system. Formal representation of employees and their interests within the framework of management was outlined as another important aspect. Here research was required but the social scientists could not envisage that radically new solutions would be found in view of previous research and the practical experience in industry.

Finally, conditions favouring personal participation was outlined as a major area for research and development. Unless further progress was made in this area other approaches seemed to be limited in scope. The researchers stressed the need to keep the programme open so that new areas could be explored on the basis of experience to be gathered and evaluated during the first phases outlined by the joint committee.

Policy matters in the initial phase of the project

No existing science policy was available to provide guidelines for the labour-management organizations when they started to explore possibilities for scientific assistance. This was the case although important national problems were involved and although financing did not seem to be the major problem.

Traditionally, social science expertise existed in the university and to a certain extent in government agencies like the Bureau of Statistics. In the latter case the expertise was limited to already well-defined community service activities. In the former case the expertise was split among academic disciplines and institutes. One could not expect these institutes to adjust to complex and long-term problem-solving in industry or other sectors of society. Not only their research tradition but also their recruitment and promotion practices and their teaching load would prevent them from entering a long-term collaborative relationship with industry. (The case would have been different for existing research centres in the field of technology.)

A small independent institute for applied social research could negotiate a research contract with the two partners in industry for the following reasons. First, it already had long-term contacts with industrial and trade union leaders. The institute had an independent position, but with the backing of a well-established academic institution to which it was attached. Second, it had already established contacts with a foreign institute – in Britain, the Tavistock Institute of Human Relations – which could help by offering the collaboration of professional social scientists with relevant experience and which could act as a neutral outsider. When the contract was settled, difficulties arose in relation to academic institutions that did not entirely favour the collaborative relationships with industry and unions. This restricted the recruitment and employment of competent people for applied research.

A stable and simple social structure made it comparatively easy for the two parties in industry to agree on a joint programme. This was based on a set of commonly agreed objectives or values which could be tested out when the programme was transformed into concrete plans for research and development. For example, values of a humanistic character, defined in terms of social and psychological needs in a work situation, were balanced against minimal requirements in terms of productivity and earnings. The researcher's integrity and values were respected in the same way as those of the other partners. This meant that each partner was free to pursue values and objectives of his own as long as this did not jeopardize the jointly defined objectives of the project. Already the identification of major problem areas to be explored represented an important step in policy-making. The establishment of a Joint Research Committee representing trade unions, employers, and researchers was another important step.

II. THE SEARCH FOR ALTERNATIVE PROBLEM-SOLVING ACTIVITIES

The Joint Research Committee was faced with two problems of allocation during the search conferences held to set up the research programme. First, in what order should the relevant problems be tackled? Second, what resources would be needed and were available for the different research activities involved? Agreement was reached on a stepwise search and employers' organizations started to work on problems of formal representation of employees in management of companies. The independent institute was granted N kr 250.000 (£35.000) for one year to analyse foreign experiences and to undertake some case studies in Norwegian companies. The institute made it clear that this was sufficient as a start, but further research for at least three more years would be needed. Decisions on this could be postponed for six months. More or less simultaneously another research group was given support to undertake descriptive studies and attitude surveys regarding participation in industry.

The independent institute made it clear that it was not willing, on the basis of existing evidence, to undertake an isolated attitude survey. The results might be misused as scientific proof that a majority of workers did not feel the need for further democratization. Alternatively some special arrangements might be supported by survey data without any reality-testing taking place. The institute agreed to study the actual experience with representative systems and simultaneously to prepare the next phase of the project.

Phase A of the project, dealing with employee representation at board level of companies, was finished in 1963. The report was worked through by the Joint National Committee before its publication in the spring of 1964 (Emery and Thorsrud, 1969b).

In 1963–4 the political situation of the country became less stable for several reasons. A coalition replaced the Labour government for a brief period and the political atmosphere became more tense because of the next general election, due to take place in 1965. The Labour Party pressed for a more radical programme on industrial democracy. A joint trade union and Labour Party committee published their preliminary recommendations, including a strengthening of representative arrangements.

The general conclusions of the researchers on the basis of phase A of the project did not, under existing conditions, support the Labour Committee recommendation. The following three points are cited from the research report:

(i) Our examination of the Norwegian firms brings into sharper focus some of the issues that emerged from the study of experiences in other European countries. In particular, there is a clear distinction between areas involving negotiation and reconciliation between different but related sources of power, and areas that seem to involve the sharing of power.

A necessary condition for the continued sharing of power is that there must be agreement on means and goals that are reconcilable with each other. Moreover, if the sharing of any source of social power is not to be disruptive of other parts of the society, then it must go hand in hand with the sharing of responsibility.

When we look at the behaviour of employee representatives on Norwegian boards, it becomes clear that although they share legally in the power of the board they find it very difficult to see how to use that power in ways that are in accord with the usual board purposes, and at the same time make a direct impact on the working life of their constituents. In most cases representatives play rather passive but loyal roles as board members. Gradually their contact and communication with other employees become weaker.

(ii) There seems to be a case for extending the area of negotiation within the firm. Works Councils and the like are potentially capable of handling a large number of problems as they arise in the concrete work setting.

The general experience is that these benefits of representational systems can be realized if they are matched by an effective management.

In general, management must recognise that the success of an enterprise depends upon how it works as a socio-technical system, not simply as a technical system with replaceable individuals added to fit.[2]

(iii) A failure to achieve democratic handling of the day-to-day problems of a company seems to undermine the work at higher levels of representation.

In most cases where a representative or consultative system

operates, the evidence seems to be that attention is primarily directed towards the first broad class of problems. These are the problems that concern the personnel division of management. The second class of problems, those relating to policy changes, major technical changes, and the like, seem to present greater difficulty for representation systems. This finding, along with other evidence, leads us to feel that the crux of the problem lies in the fact that in the day-to-day ongoing work of the enterprise there is too low a level of individual employee participation. Without some higher degree of participation at this direct level, it seems unlikely that enough interest or knowledge could be generated to sustain the sort of difficult and extended effort required to work out policies with regard to major long-term changes. Briefly, what we are suggesting is that two of the necessary conditions for the emergence of a higher level of participation are not present: these are that the individual should have more elbow-room within his job; and, second, greater responsibility for decisions affecting his job.

Several policy issues were involved in the search phase of the project. Hence the Joint National Committee agreed that one institute had to be responsible for the project, to secure long-term commitment in collaborative relationships. Complementary studies were sponsored simultaneously, but these were not covered by the policy gradually worked out by the Joint Committee. The Joint Committee also decided *what problems* should be studied. The researchers did not find problems of formal representation the most promising ones to be explored, but agreed to undertake such studies while preparations went on for the main phase of the project.

The institute responsible for the project was granted the professional right to decide what approach and what methods were relevant to the problems chosen by the committee to be covered by the research plan. In addition, principles of procedure during research and publication of results were thoroughly discussed in the Joint National Committee. The committee helped with necessary contacts in industry and unions. (Access was granted to confidential board minutes and off-the-record conversations helped to clarify the functioning of boards. Further research on board problems was initiated by these field studies.) The joint Committee also agreed to step in if problems arose during fieldwork. (This did in fact occur in later field experiments.)

Before publication took place every individual and group who had given information to be used in the report had the opportunity to check the way information had been understood and used by the researchers. The Joint Committee worked through the whole report and assisted in the diffusion of results. Researchers as well as the collaborating parties were free to draw their own conclusions from the evidence reported.

Preliminary evaluation of the different approaches to problems of industrial democracy was undertaken by all the three collaborating parties at the time when the research report was prepared by the researchers and worked through by the Joint Committee. Industrial and trade union leaders maintained somewhat different points of view regarding representative systems, although the attitudes of both sides seemed to be modified by the evidence and conclusions presented in the report from the research group. All the three parties felt free to publish their particular points of view.

Scientific evaluation in the form of professional reviewing took place when the research report was published. The collaborating parties were assured that the quality of the research was accepted by other scientists, although there were naturally differences in opinion among scientific reviewers corresponding to their special orientation. The research group could not at this point obtain from the evaluation individual academic credits. If individual qualification had been an important short-term objective for members of the research group, this would have distracted them from the major, commonly agreed objectives of the project.

Mutual evaluation and building of trust between the three collaborating parties took place in the initial phase as well as the search phase of the project. The right of each party to maintain some special interest was demonstrated. The areas of common interest had been defined and the conditions for further collaboration had been demonstrated. The Joint Committee agreed on the programme for the major phase of the project concentrating on experimental field studies. Financing for the next three years was arranged on a tripartite basis between unions, employers, and government.

III. STEPWISE EXPERIMENTAL CHANGE

Approximately 18 months had passed between the initiation of the project and the completion of the second search phase. The first plan for the main experimental phase was put forward at the end of the initiation phase. Modification of the plan took place step by step on the basis of experience gained and preliminary evaluations. The transition from phase A, dealing with formal representation, to phase B was stated in the following way:

> The manner in which employees participate in the daily work life of their companies is critical for the use they make of the mechanisms for

representation and consultation and also for their attitudes of apathy or constructive interest, of dissatisfaction or satisfaction.

The bulk of the scientific evidence suggests that the more the individual is enabled to exercise control over his task, and to relate his efforts to those of his fellows, the more likely is he to accept a positive commitment. This positive commitment shows in a number of ways, not the least of which is the release of that personal initiative and creativity that consititute the basis of a democratic climate.

However, there was no simple technique that could be applied in all industrial conditions to bring about these changes. Thus while job enlargement has proved effective in some conditions, it would be inappropriate in others; the development of autonomous work groups has been effective in some conditions, but likewise would be ineffective in others.

With this in mind, the Joint Committee considered the different sectors of industry, and decided that a start should be made in two sectors – metal-manufacturing and pulp and paper. These were considered to be strategic sectors for the national interests of unions as well as employers.

The next problem was to find within each sector a suitable plant for study. If this line of research was to be fruitful, it would be necessary not only to look at existing experience, but also to modify experimentally the conditions of personal participation and to measure resulting changes in such things as satisfaction/dissatisfaction, apathy/constructive interest, communication level, productivity and stability, continuous learning and development activities.

Experiments along these lines should be conducted in such a way that:

(i) management and employees who agreed to carry out experimental modifications of existing practices were fully informed at all stages of what was going on, and at all times felt free to urge changes in or cessation of the experiments; furthermore there should be no communication of findings without their approval;
(ii) any emergent lessons should be readily evaluated by the interested parties;
(iii) there would be a willingness to learn from these lessons, not only on the part of the company directly concerned with experimenting but also on the part of the industry as a whole.

In order that there should be a widespread willingness to learn from any emergent lessons, it was essential that the relevant leaders in management and trade unions were informed beforehand of what was being undertaken, agreed beforehand on what changes in the workplace would be relevant to their notions of industrial democracy, and agreed that the plants within which the experiments were carried out were not so exceptional as to render the results inapplicable elsewhere.

When agreement had been reached by the Joint Committee on this general policy, short-lists of potential research plants were drawn up and preliminary contacts with the managements and unions of the companies were established by the research team. During the spring of 1963 one experimental plant was chosen in metal-manufacturing and one in pulp and paper. The Joint Committee confirmed the choice and accepted the major hypotheses concerning job design that were presented by the research team, which would be basic in phase B of the project.

The final discussions in the Joint Committee before experiments started dealt with the hypotheses presented by the research group. These were hypotheses regarding design of jobs and organizational change. We cannot go into detail, but it is important to mention the general psychological requirements that were implicit in the hypotheses. They illustrated to the parties involved some of the basic values behind the project and also the potential improvements to be evaluated at some later stage. The psychological requirements related to job design were:

(i) the need for the content of a job to be reasonably demanding of the worker in terms other than sheer endurance, and yet to provide a minimum of variety (not necessarily novelty);
(ii) the need to be able to learn on the job and to go on learning – again it is a question of neither too much nor too little;
(iii) the need for some minimal area of decision-making that the individual can call his own;
(iv) the need for some minimal degree of social support and recognition in the workplace;
(v) the need for the individual to be able to relate what he does and what he produces to his social life;
(vi) the need to feel that the job leads to some sort of desirable future (not necessarily promotion).

These requirements would not be relevant only to operators on the factory floor, nor would it be possible to meet them in the same way in all work settings or for all kinds of people.

The first field experiment

The first field experiment (Marek, Lange, and Engelstad, 1964) took place in a wire-drawing mill. The principles for carrying out the experiments were agreed upon by the management of the company and by the local union, and the experimental department was selected after collaboration between the two parties and the research group. The selection was based on the type of technology, the possibility of isolating the experimental effects, and also the particular personnel problems that management and union wanted to solve (high turnover, lack of involvement, etc.).

The first phase of the field experiment consisted of a sociotechnical analysis including the following main steps:

(i) estimation of variation in inputs and outputs of materials and the main sources of variations in quality and quantity during transformation processes;
(ii) estimation of the relative importance of different variations: on the basis of the experience of operators, management, and specialists, a matrix could be produced showing the relations between variations in the system; these matrices help to identify subsystems and criteria for evaluation of critical variations. They also help to define the primary task of a department and to set up feedback arrangements;
(iii) description of formal organization;
(iv) analysis of communication networks in relation to critical variations;
(v) measurements and interviews to establish baselines for later comparison;
(vi) analysis of wage and salary systems and other job incentives;
(vii) analysis of company policies regarding training, job allocation, promotion, etc., in relation to production and marketing policies.

The second phase of the experiment was to establish, in co-operation with people in the department, a set of experimental conditions to be changed. In this case the changes were all directed towards restructuring of tasks and work-roles from a one-man/one-machine type to a group-type of work situation. Briefly what happened in this type of wire-drawing operation is this:

Thick wire is run at a very high speed through a set of reducing dies, finally emerging in a thin coil which is bundled away. The machinery required is designed in such a way that the supervision and handling involved is seen as a one-man job.

Engineers, although they have a choice in the design of the machinery, usually seem to favour the one requiring this sort of organization, i.e. one man in charge. But an examination of the workload involved shows the following pattern: most of the time the man is literally doing nothing, in fact he is probably sitting down reading a comic or paper behind his bench and out of sight of anyone else. Then suddenly the wire breaks, and he is working flat out; it is really a two-man job to get it back on, but he is the only man available. There is some handling and inspection, and a little welding, but basically the pattern of activities fails to meet the criteria of optimal workload and variety.

There is no way of modifying the old pattern in the situation of one-man/one-machine. It was necessary to redesign the work so that a group of men took group responsibility for a group of machines. In order to do this, it was necessary to make detailed calculations of the performance of each one of these machines, and of the men, to determine the appropriate workload and its variance.

Having done this, and obtained agreement from management and men for a three-month experiment, we ran into a number of difficulties. We were unable to establish all the desired experimental conditions except for a period of about two weeks. This was largely due to the fact that the men just could not believe that they were not being sold down the river by their union leadership and management – more work for less money. In the end, when they saw the results, they realized just what they could achieve through working as a group. As far as the technical side was concerned, there was practically no extra expenditure by the company on machinery or equipment, though we did manage, with difficulty, to get certain very cheap modifications introduced into the control system for stopping the machines.

We then ran into a rather peculiar problem. If the wire-drawing men were given fair payment for the production they achieved as a result of group working, they would then be among the highest-paid men in the plant. This would then raise the problem of the status of the currently highest-paid workers. It was not possible to raise everyone's pay because the plant as a whole was not producing any more, and, indeed, at the national level, this would have entailed a violation of the nationally agreed rates. (Norway, like Sweden, negotiates these at two-year intervals.)

The men in the wire mill recognized this difficulty and proposed that they be paid in time off; however, this too presented a problem, because the Employers' Federation did not want to be confronted too rapidly with a 40-hour week.

From the beginning both management and unions had been prepared to accept a significant gain on the social side, even if there had been no increase in productivity, or even if there had been a slight decrease. The hope was, of course, that there would be some extra productivity. Neither they nor we had fully realized the difficulties created by extra productivity. The problem has still not been resolved, though the company has set up groups of its own people to get to work in other departments and possibly move them in the same direction. In retrospect we can see a number of reasons why this has not yet occurred.

Some policy issues related to the first field experiment

Let us first summarize some policy issues at *company level.*

First, the objectives of the local experiment were agreed upon formally between management, union, and researchers. However, the implications of the experiment could not be envisaged clearly by the local people and in reality there was no joint involvement and commitment to follow up the experiment, to make a joint evaluation, and possibly to change the local policies. The researchers were not sufficiently aware of the time and resources necessary to build up the local conditions for policy-making as a learning process. The local people looked at the experiment as an isolated event relating it to the national situation and not so much to learning and change at local level. The local union backed the Trade Union Council and management supported the Employers' Association in their policies to get local experiments started. The local conditions and possible consequences were not really evaluated.

Second, the necessary conditions for joint local evaluation were not created early enough to establish the roles and the social learning process required to achieve a diffusion of results at company level. The researchers had not developed a strategy by which they could move from a set of roles necessary to get the experiment under way to a different set of roles necessary to achieve evaluation and local initiative and responsibility for continuous learning and policy-making. Both management and union leaders at local level looked on the experiment in much the same way as they would look on a technological experiment. They found it difficult to accept that they had both the ability and the obligation to share in the evaluation of results in relation to the existing conditions. It is important to note that local leaders had no other experiments to use as models for their own evaluations.

The conditions for scientific evaluation of the experiment were far from perfect, but were sufficiently good for the social scientists to claim strong support for the central hypothesis that job design could be related to the main objectives of the project. Some tensions developed in the research group in relation to scientific evaluation and the future academic status of the members, but this did not distract the group from its main task, namely to produce a research report for evaluation by the Joint National Committee.

Let us now consider some policy issues at the *national level.* The Joint Committee could well understand the limitations of the situation at company level. Consequently these limitations did not distract the committee from making the necessary evaluations and reallocation of resources necessary for further experimentation.

The objectives and underlying values of the project had been operationally defined in the first experiment and could now be re-evaluated by the Joint Committee. A decision was made that further experimentation should take place according to the original plan. The interrelation between policies for democratization and policies for training and education, on the one hand, and the settlement of wages and work conditions, on the other, was now better understood. Policy discussions in these other areas started and have since led to changes at the national level, at least to some extent under the influence of the Industrial Democracy Project. If policy-making is a learning process, one must not expect it to be simple or limited to a single sector. This is certainly the case when science policy and large organizations are involved.

The principles governing the stepwise experimental change process had been demonstrated and were accepted by the Joint Committee. Representatives of management and labour were reassured that the alternatives proposed by the research group were promising although they were not easy to realize, particularly if management and employee representatives did not play a very active role in the change process. This involvement would give the main labour and management organizations a chance to be fully informed. It would enable them to exercise leadership and control, but there were strong indications already in the first field experiment that decentralization of organizational control would have to take place if the ideas behind the project were to be realized.

The second field experiment

At the time when the first field experiment had reached the stage of local evaluation and diffusion, a second experiment was started in the pulp and paper industry. The Joint Committee helped with the selection of the plant and the introduction on the management and union side. At a very early point local management and union explored, *together* with the research group, the basic ideas behind the project and the possible consequences. There was mutual agreement on central issues – for instance, the need for training at all levels and for improvement of the communication network. On one central point however there seemed to be disagreement, namely the role of the first-line supervisor, which management had recently tried to strengthen in order to improve production control on the shop floor. The leading union representative maintained that this was probably a step in the wrong direction, since it would reduce the motivation and ability of operators to play a responsible role.

The first analysis of the plant revealed the following characteristics. The main task was information-handling requiring a high degree of technological skill. A large range of information flows had to be handled not only within each shift group and department, but also between shifts and departments. To improve this situation a reallocation of responsibilities seemed to be necessary between supervisors, key operators, and assistant operators. On-the-job training would be crucial to achieve this, but important changes were also needed in the technical basis for measurements and communication. Considerable effort was spent in selecting appropriate points for instrumentation and communication links to be developed, so that operators along the total process could contribute to summarizing information and exercising control. Simultaneously, training needs were analysed and the role of the foreman was studied. He appeared to be fully occupied; however, when the activity was viewed from the technical side, the key information flows were by-passing him.

The research group developed an action programme, in collaboration with operators, supervisors, and specialists. Specific conditions were defined to achieve a higher degree of sociotechnical optimization. The main conditions were related to information systems, training programmes for operators and supervisors, job rotation arrangement, bonus on quality, decentralized maintenance, and transfer of supervisors to boundary control (rather than intradepartmental control). At this stage of the experiment an important event took place. A joint meeting of operators, supervisors, managers, and union representatives decided that a local action committee should take over the main responsibility for the experiment. The research group was to withdraw to a consultative role and to assist in measuring the results. Only if this took place could the four major steps outlined for the experiment be realized. These were:

(i) information to everyone involved;
(ii) involvement on a voluntary basis;
(iii) commitment to a stepwise change programme;
(iv) joint action to achieve social and technological change.

After the local action committee took over, a number of significant changes were carried out in the experimental pulp department in 1965–6. Significant improvements could be measured in terms of production control, local learning, and initiative for technological change (Engelstad, 1968). However, the company was hit by severe problems in the international paper market and several aspects of the change programme were given a lower priority than immediate action that had to be taken for the company to survive. A major problem appeared in terms of insecurity among groups of personnel. A new company policy on supervision and production management did not emerge quickly enough to reinforce the learning and change processes that had started on the shop floor. Several of the improvements in job design and organization development deteriorated, although the basic ideas seemed to have taken root in the company.

Three years after the initiation of the second field experiment, the company and the local union agreed to proceed to a new experiment in the paper factory. In this case the role of the foreman was brought up for analysis immediately. In fact a decision was made to run two paper machines without the traditional shift foremen, who were transferred to other tasks. After one year of experience with this system different levels of management and union have decided to apply the principles of partly autonomous work groups throughout the company. It is still too early to evaluate the consequences of this decision.

At the national level, the experiences from the second field experiment led to a decision in the Joint Committee to accept the responsibility for two more experiments and the prolongation of the research programme. The third experiment took place in a small assembly plant and the fourth one in a large electrochemical enterprise with a number of plants in different parts of Norway and also abroad.

Some policy issues related to the second field experiment

First, the link was strengthened between local experimentation and a national policy in a special sector as it emerged in the Joint Committee on social science research on industrial democracy. The experience from the first experiment was transferred to the second – initially through personal contacts to central level. Gradually, elements of policy were explicitly formulated. One such element was the protection of field sites, for a limited period of time, from outside interference caused by policies in areas other than social research. Typically some aspects of national wage and salary policy and certain principles of job simplification and specialization of training went contrary to the principles tested out in the field experiments. Co-ordination of different policies had to be postponed until experimental evidence could be produced. Another element of explicit policy was related to the local responsibility for experimentation and diffusion of results. The constitution of the local action committee and the gradual withdrawal of the research team were accepted as specific policy in further research.

In retrospect it can be observed that the stepwise change and the corresponding evaluation of results was a basic condition for local development as well as for policy-making at central level. At the same time the evaluation process was threatening to some local leaders as well as to members of the research team. Exposing success or failure in certain respects could easily be interpreted as rewarding or punishing individuals.

Second, it was demonstrated that a matrix of roles had to be developed to fit the changing requirements of experimentation and policy-making. Introduction of a new policy of organization at company level was dependent on mutual backing by management as well as union, just as mutual backing at national level was a precondition for local experiments. Change at one level of the organization, i.e. supervisor or operator, had to be supported by corresponding changes in organizational roles at other levels. The same applied to different levels of trade union representatives. The changes in roles on each side and at different levels were quite likely to have consequences on the power relationships between different roles and different organizations. The policy implications of such changes were observed at national level and the consequences had to be evaluated in relation to the basic goals set up for the research and development programme. In retrospect it can be observed that management was given more freedom to act at local level although this might have endangered the bargaining position of the Employers' Association in certain respects. Likewise the local trade union started to exercise initiative in such a way that it might over time change the relative influence of central headquarters. In general it seems as if the research and learning at local level generated a consciousness in policy matters that started to flow upwards in both labour and management organizations. Obviously policy-making in relation to research cannot be isolated from policies in other areas. Any change in policy seems to imply a change in resource allocation for the realization of certain plans or programmes. This automatically has consequences for allocation of resources, for programmes and plans in other sectors.

The third and fourth field experiments

This paper has outlined in some detail the first two experiments in order to illustrate in concrete terms how policy-making and local change are interrelated. Before we analyse the policy issues of the final phases of this research project we shall briefly mention field experiments number three and four.

The third experiment took place in a small subsidiary assembly plant producing electrical panel heaters. The experimental conditions were fairly easy to define and measurements could be compared between this plant and a corresponding department located in a nearby city. Routine operations on the production line in the major factory were reorganized within three partly autonomous work groups. Individual incentives and specialized jobs were substituted for group bonus and job rotation. Production planning and simple maintenance tasks were decentralized. After a ten-week experiment and two years of follow-up, clear evidence could be presented in terms of improved fulfilment of the basic psychological job requirements referred to earlier in this paper. The level of productivity and earnings increased substantially (Thorsrud and Emery, 1969b). A major outcome of this experiment was that the new system of work organization spread to another department in the same plant without any assistance from the research group. Further diffusion into the main plant has not yet occurred, mainly because the experimental results have not been evaluated and integrated into the personnel and organizational policy of the company.

The fourth field experiment took place in a highly automated fertilizer plant belonging to one of the major industrial enterprises in Norway. The principles of job design and organizational development tested out in the first three experiments were applied to the new field site. A local action committee was linked to central headquarters of the corporation and to corresponding trade union bodies. An intensive action programme was carried out in terms of job design, integration of process operation and maintenance, training activity at several levels and within different sectors of the organization. Wage and salary systems were changed and supervisory and specialist roles redefined. After a brief period of experimental testing of the new principles of work organization, an evaluation of preliminary results led to a decision to start four new experimental plants in the same enterprise. This does not mean that a systematic change in the personnel and organization policy of the whole corporation has been realized. However, explicit policy declarations from top management and trade union officials have been made to initiate such a change. This corporation and the corresponding unions have considerable impact and parallel responsibilities in national policy-making. A leading executive from the corporation and a trade union leader who played a major role in starting the fourth experiment have been elected members of the Joint National Committee. This means that local and national policy-making has to be integrated. In some cases this can speed up the policy-making process – in some instances it can slow it down. At the moment there are several policy issues emerging from field experiments number three and four.

The major issues are related to the evaluation and diffusion of research results at national level. We shall therefore comment briefly on these phases of the project before we summarize our final points regarding policy.

IV. EVALUATION AND DIFFUSION OF RESULTS AT THE NATIONAL LEVEL

When the research report on the four field experiments was finished in 1968 and given clearance at local union and company level, the Joint

Research Committee was invited to make decisions regarding the publishing and utilization of the results. Some main results and some conclusions had already been discussed in union and management groups and among specialists. The Joint Committee decided that the report should be published with the support of the Trade Union Council and the National Confederation of Employers. A special council, which had been established two years earlier (National Council on Participation in Industry), was asked to take the responsibility for diffusion and utilization of the results. Training seminars were set up for managers and specialists and for trade union representatives. The two main organizations in industry started activities to prepare their members to be able to apply the new principles of job design and organizational development. A joint statement was issued regarding the initiation of a series of new experiments with the objective of testing the new principles under new sets of social and technological conditions. Several groups of specialists, mainly in training, in industrial engineering, and in wage and salary systems started to explore the consequences of the Industrial Democracy Project for their own professional principles and practices.

It is obviously too early to judge the effects of this phase of the project, but several main issues can be observed.

Policy issues related to evaluation and diffusion of results

In the first instance, the main sponsors acted as guardians to protect the results of the project from co-optation by special interest groups. They also warned their members that although the new principles of organization represented a promising approach to problems of industrial democracy they could not be applied as isolated techniques. Significant changes in related fields had to be introduced if desirable results were to be achieved.

Further, the evaluation of results from the project within each of the main organizations in industry led to corresponding evaluations in related policies. Decentralization of certain aspects of contract bargaining has been considered. A gradual change-over from individual incentive systems to fixed salary rates combined with local group bonuses seems to be taking place. Time-study techniques and rigid job specification applied to improve the efficiency of individual workers are being judged critically. More emphasis is put on joint optimization of social and technological factors at group and departmental level. Collective bargaining now takes into consideration the integration of industrial training and adult education with other conditions for personal participation. The organizational structure of unions is discussed also in relation to the democratization of the workplace. It is however much too early to judge how far the integration of policies worked out by the Joint Research Committee will be supported by and integrated into the more complex structure of policies controlled by the labour and management organizations and by government.

The scientific evaluation of the research project has become more active since the main research report (Thorsrud and Emery, 1969b) was published and the diffusion of results has become widespread. Constructive criticism has helped the research group and the sponsors to be aware of the limitations and new possibilities of their programme. Closer contacts have been established with academic research and educational centres. The student revolt and current criticism of any research linked to established organizations has occasionally made it difficult to differentiate political from scientific criticism.

On the whole, the project has not been subject to such political pressure or criticism that the integrity of the social scientists has been endangered. The individual academic credits earned by members of the research group have been smaller than if they had been engaged in research directed by traditional rules set by separate academic disciplines. The interdisciplinary character of the project and the involvement in significant human and social affairs has made it not too difficult for the research team to remain task-oriented. The evaluation process which we have assumed to be crucial to any change in social policies has occasionally caused tensions within the research group. Since gradually pressure has declined for the researchers to be more or less continuously involved in fieldwork and since more time can be allocated to theoretical work, these tensions may decrease.

V. RE-ALLOCATION OF RESOURCES

If policy-making can be described as a learning process, we would expect a reallocation of resources to take place on the basis of stepwise experimentation and evaluation. In 1969 when there was about one year left of the existing research plan and corresponding funds, the collaborating parties started to discuss a reallocation and continuation of a broader programme. In the meantime a special project within the same general framework had started in the Norwegian merchant navy, with the approval of the Joint Committee, but financed by the users. Requests had also come from school authorities to the research group pointing to the interrelations between industrial democracy and the democratization of educational systems.

The research group worked out a draft for a revised research programme containing the following main items:

continued organizational research to explore the wider theoretical and practical aspects of the field experiments carried out so far;
continued work on methods and techniques within the general framework of sociotechnical theory;
research and follow-up of the strategy for diffusion of social science results.
A possible transfer of research methods and theory to other areas than industry and shipping was considered, but limited resources and the need for further verification made the researchers hesitant to become very active in other fields. Preliminary studies were about to start in education.

The Joint National Committee discussed the new research proposal in several meetings and each one of the major collaborating parties judged the plans separately. There was common agreement on the major aspects of the programme, particularly that the necessary conditions must be created for the interdisciplinary research group to be kept together. If this did not occur, one would expect most members of the team to join academic institutes, where safer career lines were open. Some parts of further financing could easily be arranged since a widespread demand for social science assistance now existed in industry and related fields, and a distinctive competence in the research group had been demonstrated. However, the Joint Committee agreed that government should now take a greater responsibility for financing a broader research programme to be allocated to the Work Research Institute in Oslo. Representatives of the committee met representatives of government at top level, and early in 1970 a special *ad hoc* group put forward a new programme and plans for financing for a new three-year period. Academic institutes are now involved in the new programme for the purpose of increasing the recruitment of qualified researchers and stimulating similar research in these institutes, a task that can well be combined with their educational and research tasks.

The Joint Committee has also discussed how the main industrial and trade union organizations can strengthen their own staff to be professionally equipped for active collaboration with social scientists and outside specialists.

SOME POLICY ISSUES IN RETROSPECT

Many social scientists may feel this paper to be peripheral to what they consider to be the major issues in social science policy. They will argue that a policy discussion should deal more exclusively with the broader issues such as the objectives, the long-term planning, and the allocation of resources for the mobilization of the social sciences. They may regard as misleading the use of an applied research project to demonstrate major aspects of policy-making in the social sciences. In my view, on the contrary, one of the main problems in social science policy is the balance between applied and fundamental or basic research.

The tendency to keep policy discussions in general terms has made the author sceptical after having listened over the last ten years to hundreds of so-called policy discussions among management representatives in industry. If any conclusions are reached, they tend to be so general that almost no one can disagree. Consequently they have no impact upon choice between alternative lines of action. If specific details are to be related to policy, it is frequently stated that such details will have to be judged in view of the existing conditions in each case.

Less is learned about the policy of a company from analysing policy statements regarding the future than from looking into its recent history. If one can find *why* the company *did not* choose certain lines of action, one gets an impression of where it is going or not going in the future when choice is open. Radical reallocation of its resources is usually slow. The criteria the firm uses to evaluate its past and present activities indicate what objectives it is going to pursue. Finally, if one can find what aspects of its environment and what coalitions and competitors the firm takes into account for future adjustments, one can also conclude something about its policy. In fact, we are back to the point of view that policy-making can be understood as a complex learning and adjustment process over time.

In retrospect these are some of the policy issues that have occurred and have been dealt with in a particular social science project over the last eight years:

(i) Policy-making in the social sciences can be described only if we accept that we are dealing with a highly complex process taking place over time and including many interest groups. Policy-making always includes choice between alternative plans of action according to value criteria. But value criteria have meaning only in terms of the more specific principles governing choice between alternative ways of reaching goals. The alternative ways and goals can only be specified in relation to assessments of available and potential resources. Even when such assessments can be made without initiating too great a struggle for power among interest groups no responsible social scientist can guarantee specific outcomes of special programmes. If this were possible, no research would in fact be required. We therefore look at policy-making as a complex learning process. The learning starts with preliminary clarification of a problem area. It proceeds with a search for alternative problem-solving activities allocated experimentally to collaborating partners in a research and development process. A stepwise experimentation and predefined evaluation of research approaches and results have to take place at the end of each distinctive phase. A certain degree of diffusion of results has to be arranged before all-over evaluation can be made of approaches, and methods, and results as a basis for reallocation of resources. In retrospect a policy-making process can look much more systematic than it has actually been – much more orderly than it can actually be. Social science in contrast to many other activities consists of indeterminate tasks with indeterminate outcomes. Rather than striving for the establishment of well-defined science policies, we should concentrate on the conditions under which policy-making can start or develop over time.

(ii) Social science policy does not exist in a vacuum. Policy-making in related fields will sometimes speed up and sometimes slow down or block developments in social science. Social scientists have to create collaborative relationships with representatives of other groups to be tried out stepwise over time. Avoidance of a monolithic power structure in social science as well as among collaborating parties will be a precondition for development of a constructive division of tasks and responsibilities between scientists and other groups. A pluralistic model for social science organization follows from an analysis of the different task structures and collaborative relationships required for different kinds of research programmes. The distinctive competence of researchers in academic institutes is influenced by their educational responsibilities within special disciplines. The competence of researchers in institutes involved in applied research will be influenced by their long-term responsibility for interdisciplinary professional facilitation of social change.

(iii) Experiences from a long-term social science programme shows the distinction between theoretical and applied research to be misleading. Allocation of resources for social science must therefore be made in such a way that applied research will periodically be concentrated on theoretical work and sometimes on data-gathering or experimentation in the field.

(iv) The evaluation process – a necessary part of any policy-making process over time – demands different criteria to be worked out for different phases of a research programme. Different roles and interest groups must be involved in evaluation of different phases. If, for instance, applied research is judged only on the basis of achievement in predefined problem-solving, it will tend to develop towards consulting work. If research is judged only on the basis of academic criteria set by separate disciplines, it will tend to be isolated from social life and from the policy-making processes in which different interest groups will usually be involved.

(v) Policy-making, like complex learning in actual life situations, will only create a certain degree of stability for a limited period of time. Policy-making in the social sciences should be kept open to changes in the social sciences as well as in the social scene.

Notes

[1] This formulation (policy-making as a learning process) emerged in discussions with Philip G. Herbst.

[2] This has been formulated as the principle of joint optimization. Briefly this states that the objectives of an enterprise are unlikely to be best met by optimizing conditions for either the social or the technical system at the expense of the other. The best fit between the two systems, and the best performance, are likely to involve less than the best possible conditions for both systems.

References

EMERY, F. E., and THORSRUD, E., *Form and Content in Industrial Democracy*, Tavistock Publications, London, 1969a.

MAREK, J., LANGE, K., and ENGELSTAD, P. H., Industrial Democracy Project, Wire-Drawing Mill of the Christiania Spigerverk. *Report 1*, Institute for Industrial Research, NTH, 1964.

ENGELSTAD, P. H., The Hunsfos Experiment. Work Research Institutes, Oslo, 1968.

THORSRUD, E., and EMERY, F. E., *Mot en ny bedriftsorganisasjon*. (*Towards New Organizational Forms in Enterprise*.) Tanum, Oslo, 1969b.

Interchapter

In the previous session, the discussions were concerned with the relationship between the policy-maker and the social scientist at the macro-level; in this session there was a more detailed focus on the forms of relationship developed within one specific research project. The example was the Industrial Democracy Project that had been carried out in Norway. Professor Thorsrud discussed some of the implications of the use of a collaborative-style relationship, i.e. one in which the researchers and policy-makers, in this case employers and trade union officials, are jointly responsible for decisions regarding the research programme, its evaluation, and the diffusion of the results.

Thorsrud regards the policy-making process as a learning process, and researchers working with policy-makers in this collaborative-type relationship are involved in a mutual learning process. When we look back from any point in time there appears to be a logical, orderly process in which we can pinpoint stages of this learning process, but we know that this picture is totally unrealistic. Similarly, policies appear to be reached through some ordered and logical process, although in practice many policies are articulated only after decisions and actions have been taken. In the Industrial Democracy Project the collaborative relationship between the researchers and the client is a mutual learning process from which policy-making emerges. Hence it does not fit the traditional model which assumes that a policy-making procedure must be formally established into which advice from social scientists can be fitted.

In applied or consultancy work with industry or any other client, a social science researcher must avoid being placed in the position of being asked to do things that he is not competent to do. Clients will often cast him in the specialist's role, as the teacher who can tell them what to do; however, the nature of the collaborative relationship has to be carefully explored with the client to ensure that he will be prepared to accept the framework of joint decision-making. This is particularly important in deciding upon experimental changes, and even more in setting up criteria for evaluating whether these are the results of the whole research exercise or of small experimental projects. The diffusion of the results depends upon a common understanding between client and researcher. For this sort of research to have any value, both to the client and to the 'academic world', the general approach to evaluation and diffusion of the research results must be considered at the very outset. The criteria for evaluating, and the means of diffusing, the results will vary considerably for the client and for the academic world, but the results of the research can only be meaningful if the client and the researcher jointly agree on criteria for evaluating it before the study has progressed into the experimental stage.

As scientists, we have tremendous power and influence – we have resources in terms of knowledge and we have privileged access to students, and this lays great responsibility upon us. As it becomes easier for us to become involved in the policy-making process, we must self-critically examine our present posture and the direction in which we are to go. We can stick to traditional work within the social sciences, keeping to our own disciplines and staying within the universities. We can involve ourselves in building social science capability into those organizations, particularly service organizations, which could usefully establish 'in-house' social science research. Or we can enter into long-term engagements with clients, but this is best done by professional institutes of applied social science research.

This naturally led on to discussion of the appropriate forms of organization for this sort of applied research and the appropriate training for students who wish to be applied researchers. These questions were taken up again later and are discussed in Chapter 6.

Returning to the topic of the relationship between the researcher and the policy-maker, it was pointed out that the tone of the discussions during the previous session was decidedly one of pessimism, whereas Thorsrud had been able to introduce a note of optimism into the debate.

Three factors caused the pessimism of the previous session: (a) social scientists experience difficulty in locating those policy-makers whose area of influence corresponds to their own area of competence; (b) there is no vehicle on the policy-making side to transfer knowledge from the social scientist to the policy-maker; (c) the researchers do not have sufficient say in the selection of problems that the client wishes to solve and in the presentation of the results of the research to those whom it concerns.

In the Industrial Democracy Project these three problems were overcome largely through the relationship that was developed between the research team and the policy-makers.

While this collaborative-style relationship with its mutual learning process would seem to have many advantages for the utilization of social science research, social scientists should not rigidly follow one particular model but give very serious consideration to how the findings of each individual applied research project may be utilized. As our discussions during this conference have shown, social scientists and policy-makers may relate to one another in many different ways. Our knowledge of our disciplines has grown because we use scientific methods, we give great thought to our own methodology, and we report it in detail. Our knowledge of the process of utilization of research will grow likewise only if we treat this as a scientific topic, give great thought to its methodology, and report it in detail. This implies honest reporting of what failed as well as what was successful.

4 Research and public policy

Lessons from economics

Andrew Shonfield

Social science is a blanket term covering many activities and several discrete and identifiable disciplines. The involvement of social science with public policy has not been uniform and certain areas have grown closer to and more entwined with the policy sector than others. In Western Europe and the USA, economics more than any other social science discipline has gained the ear of the policy-makers, both through its influence in established government agencies such as budget bureaux and treasuries and through formal advisory mechanisms such as the US Council of Economic Advisors. Indeed, political problems are frequently viewed as economic problems to the extent that social variables are often cast misleadingly in economic terms.

In this chapter, Andrew Shonfield puts forward some reasons for the close involvement of economics with the business of policy formation – first, it operates within a comprehensive theoretical system which in principle links all relevant variables in its area of study and, second, it deals with what he terms 'manageable aggregates' of social data. The other social science disciplines will only relate more closely to public policy if they move in these directions, and one way to achieve this is through the development of social indicators.

Social indicators currently excite a large amount of attention from both the social science community and the political sector. Shonfield examines the difficult theoretical criteria that must be satisfied by any successful indicator system and discusses some operational difficulties likely to be involved in applying them. In conclusion, he considers the task of establishing a system of indicators is a long-term one, but nevertheless it seems probable that through such a process the wider influence of social science thinking on the establishment of policy goals would be substantially increased.

Andrew Shonfield is Chairman of the British Social Science Research Council. He is Director General Designate of the Royal Institute of International Affairs, London, where he was formerly Director of Studies (1961–8). Focusing on economics in its wider social context, Shonfield's major publications include *Modern Capitalism* (1965), *Attack on World Poverty* (1960), and *British Economic Policy since the War* (1959).

ECONOMICS AND POLICY

With the growth of government patronage of social science, a large number of social scientists have come to spend a great deal of their time trying to anticipate impending changes in public policy. It is no bad thing that their political sensibilities are aroused in this way. One cannot fail to be impressed by the speed with which governments in the advanced West European countries can nowadays assemble a team of able and well-equipped researchers to investigate some urgent problem, as a preliminary to legislative or administrative action. The tempo is almost American.

However, governments themselves are not invariably particularly quick or percipient in identifying the research problems that are relevant to policy choices. Indeed, social science research is unlikely to be fully effective while it is held at arm's length and treated as a kind of servicing organization to be used after the main decisions have been taken. If social scientists were accepted as an integral element in the process of formulating the objectives of policy and in determining the pattern of priorities, the chances are that their researches would be more closely related to changing policy requirements. There is such a rapid rate of obsolescence of particular social problems and such a high rate of growth of new ones that exceptional demands are likely to be made on scientific researchers working in this field. Delay in identifying the relevant questions that lend themselves to scientific investigation within the appropriate time-scale can be costly.

The evidence suggests that of all the social sciences economics is most involved in the business of policy formulation. It is worth asking whether, and if so how, the other social sciences might achieve a similar result. The remainder of this paper addresses itself to that question.

It is characteristic of economics that it sets the actual terms in which questions of policy related to the subject are posed. Economic policy is recognized as a matter for economists, not only in the sense that they are invited to provide expert advice on the means to be employed to achieve specified ends – that would apply to other social scientists in their respective spheres – but in arguing about the ends themselves. The point can best be made by considering a particular policy objective, e.g. price stability. If it were treated as a simple imperative, as it has been treated at various times by governments in the past, then the policy-makers would need the services of the economist only to advise about the choice of means – how much taxation, what level of interest rates, and so on. But it is nowadays generally recognized that the instruments used to secure price stability are very likely to affect other objectives of economic policy – a high rate of growth, for example, or full employment. Expert economic advice is therefore needed right from the start of the policy-making process.

Essentially, its function is to supply guidance on the 'trade-off' between the mutually competitive elements in a policy. The kind of question that ultimately has to be asked of the policy-maker is: how big an increase in prices are you willing to trade against some additional growth in the real national product? The aim of the various calculations that are made in the process of answering this question is to balance the various objectives of policy against one another until, to use economists' jargon, the 'marginal value' of the fulfilment of each one of them is equal. If the situation were unequal at the margin, that would imply that a higher total satisfaction of policy objectives could be secured by transferring resources from some activity showing a lower return to one showing a higher return. To achieve the theoretically perfect 'trade-off' requires a lot of these imaginary bargains, measuring a variety of costs and benefits against one another. A cabinet debating its economic policy would be very foolish if it failed to involve professional economists in this process.

The question then is whether economics is of its essence a unique case or whether it is reasonable to look forward to analogous status in the sphere of public affairs for the other social sciences which are equally germane to government policy.

One possible answer is that economics has a peculiar relationship with politics – it is a subject with such a powerful doctrinal appeal to politicians that they take its dicta exceptionally seriously. This was Keynes's view, which he developed with a fine flourish in the concluding section of *The General Theory of Employment, Interest, and Money*:

> Practical men, who believe themselves to be quite exempt from any intellectual influences, are usually the slaves of some defunct economist. Madmen in authority, who hear voices in the air, are distilling their frenzy from some academic scribbler of a few years back. I am sure that the power of vested interests is vastly exaggerated compared with the gradual encroachment of ideas. Not, indeed, immediately, but after a certain interval – for in the field of economic and political philosophy there are not many who are influenced by new theories after they are 25 or 30 years of age, so that the ideas which civil servants and politicians and even agitators apply to current events are not likely to be the newest (Keynes, 1936).

Although there is plainly something in this, it would only explain why economic theory has for long had such a powerful *ideological* influence; that was as true in the mid-1930s when Keynes was writing this passage as it is today. But what is different between now and then is the greatly increased scientific use of economics as an instrument of empirical measurement. Today any government of an advanced country in the Western world will normally make the attempt to measure in advance the economic consequences of various policy proposals which it is trying to trade off against one another. The measurement may not always be very subtle and in the end, no doubt, as in all the affairs of government, the impulses and personal preferences of the governors play a part. But there is at least an established procedure that is gone through – even if, in the end, 'the defunct economist' wins out against the modern econometrician.

No comparably systematic effort is made to bring the other social sciences into the business of formulating social policy. Their expertise is pretty well confined to the elaboration of more efficient means. This is partly because social aims tend to be viewed as discrete items, and so the amalgam of items selected by a politician or someone else to make up a policy is thought of as being determined very largely by individual temperament and choice. There is no common measure of benefit or cost that can be employed to secure some degree of objective judgement between them. It is true of course that a social programme will usually set out to secure a broad consistency among the main objectives to be pursued. However, the consistency sought is usually a matter of the appropriate moral stance associated with a particular set of ideals, rather than an operational requirement imposed by the nature of data subjected to scientific analysis. One catches an occasional glimpse of what the alternative process could be like when a social scientist is able to introduce a body of theory as a guide to policy, imposing a certain consistent pattern on the choices to be made, and thus setting the terms in which certain non-economic decisions are made – in the manner of an economist. An interesting example of the latter was the report by Daniel Moynihan in 1965, when he was Assistant Secretary in the US Department of Labor, on the crucial place of the unstable negro family structure in the development of race relations in the United States. President Johnson adopted a large-scale programme of reforms based on the theories about the functioning of American negro society underlying the report, explicitly designed 'to strengthen the family, to create conditions under which most parents will stay together . . .' (Lyons, 1969). But this kind of event is rare and when it occurs the body of professional social scientists are by no means uniformly gratified. They tend to see it in terms of a sleight of hand by which one of their number has managed arbitrarily to capture and use the power of a politician – in the sort of way that Lysenko used Stalin.

H. W. Riecken has suggested that not only economics but also psychology must be distinguished from the rest of the social sciences as regards their influence on policy formulation. 'Both are considerably more active in the day-to-day affairs of the world than the other social sciences are and are more successful in applying their methods, techniques and knowledge to practical problems.' And he suggests that the reason is that 'both are future-oriented rather than past-oriented and both are concerned with prediction or control' (Riecken, 1969). However, this does not seem to me to be the crucial factor that makes for the characteristic type of involvement that economics has in contemporary policy formulation – and I suspect that putting it in the same bracket with psychology may serve to confuse the issue. Indeed, Riecken himself makes the point later on in the same paragraph as that from which I have quoted, that the typical method of psychologists is to proceed 'by manipulating the various features of the stimulus situation', and that economists rarely have an opportunity to carry out experiments in a comparable fashion. The truth is that the methodology of experimental psychology distinguishes it sharply from all the other social sciences. If the results that it obtains influence the decisions of governments and other social organizations, it is for the same reason that the results obtained by experimental work in the natural sciences do so. The simple point is that hypotheses that can be validated by controlled experiments have a different status from those which cannot.

There are two characteristic features of economics at its present stage of development which, I suspect, largely account for its peculiar role in policy formulation. The first has already been indicated: it operates within a comprehensive theoretical system which, at any rate in principle, purports to cover the relationships between all the relevant phenomena in its field of study. For example an economist who made a recommendation to the British government about a change in the money supply would not be surprised to be asked how this might affect the level of employment in the building industry in a district in the north of Scotland. He might not be able to answer the question offhand, but he would be able to show how the connection between the two phenomena would work. A sociologist advising on a proposed change in the structure of some institution, say, the primary schools, would not expect to be able to supply answers to a lot of questions about how this was likely to affect the operation of authority in other institutions, e.g. the factories or the law courts. No doubt some intelligent guesses could be made, but the sociologist would not be able to call in aid a well-established analytical framework that would show how the causal nexus between these disparate phenomena was likely to function. That is not to claim that if a number of economists were asked the first question they would produce a unanimous answer; they might well give different weights to various factors in the final equation.

But there would be a wide measure of agreement on the main structural features of the system as a whole.

The second factor that tends to give economics an advantage compared with the other social sciences is its greater facility in measuring *manageable aggregates* of social data. What I mean by 'manageable' is the kind of information that a practical man exercising power can use to change or to manage some segment of the social system. As Riecken perceptively remarks: 'By fixing attention upon variables about which no action can be taken most sociologists provide theoretical and explanatory structure that have neither interest nor promise for the social problem-solver because he cannot use them as handles or levers' (Riecken, op. cit., p. 110). It is not the fact that economics is 'future-oriented' and given to making predictions that gives it its special character. Making predictions, more particularly short-term predictions, is one of its important contributions to the management of society, and although some of these predictions are very imperfect their quality and usefulness steadily increase. But even if economics were less successful in this kind of forecasting, its place in the policy-making apparatus of government would still be crucial. And that is because of its ability to express in verifiable units of measurement the situation *as of now*. This means (a) that it can, by using its large accumulation of measured data from the past, plot underlying trends; and (b) that it can establish fairly precise conditions for the validation or rejection of hypotheses about the further development of these trends in the future. In fact the most useful thing that the discipline has done, which would alone justify the attention paid to it by policy-makers, is to create a large array of economic indicators.

MOVES TOWARDS SOCIAL INDICATORS

This is the decisive difference between economics and the other social sciences as a policy-making instrument. If there is any one thing that could help to relate social science research more closely to public policy, it is the rapid development of efficient social indicators. The recent spate of work in this field, especially that done under the leadership of the US Department of Health, Education, and Welfare, reflects the sense of inadequacy of many of the social scientists who have been involved in the work of government. They have found that the simplest questions about the trend of criminal behaviour, or about health and morbidity, or about differences in the welfare of minority groups elude them.

The initial response to the evidence of this glaring deficiency in social policy-making was to think in terms of a comprehensive Social Account to complement the National Income Accounts (see notably Gross, 1966). It very soon became evident that our understanding of the workings of the social system was quite inadequate to establish a set of relationships, analogous to the national income model, between the input of social resources and the output of social products. For a start, we do not have any kind of measure of the global totals, whether of input or output. There is therefore no way of achieving comprehensive itemization of what one is trying to measure; one can never say – here are some of the main components of the system and what is left over makes up a residuum of a certain order of magnitude. Then there is the problem of identifying individual items. If one takes an input like education and tries to trace its flow through the social system, one finds straight away that there are enormous difficulties about separating it from other factors with which the educational process is irretrievably associated – the health of pupils, their home conditions, the cultural activities of the community to which they belong, and so on. This is typical of social inputs in general. There is in fact almost unlimited scope for 'double-counting' of a given input which is present in some degree under a number of different headings used in the analysis. The same type of problem applies to the analysis of output. It is true that there are similar conceptual difficulties in certain kinds of economic analysis, notably in cost-benefit studies, about avoiding the 'double-counting' of inputs. But the methods of economic analysis contain a number of built-in checks against this kind of mistake. They are absent in social analysis. The preliminary condition for setting up a comprehensive Social Account is a satisfactory theory of how the system works. The causal connections between the various parts of society are in fact so obscure that it is hardly likely that this condition will soon be met.

An alternative course is to concentrate on the measurement of social 'output', without first trying to solve the problem of identifying causal connections within the system. The field of study in this case would be the delineation of significant social change. Social indicators of the type that would serve this purpose would not have a predictive function. The sense in which the social changes that they measure could be said to be 'significant' would simply be that these changes had been singled out for special attention because of the relevance that they were *deemed* to have to the making of policy decisions. In other words, the people concerned with decisions about social policy – and that might in a democratic society include a large part of the population – believed that their arguments could be supported or contradicted by the evidence brought together in the various indicators.

There are however some genuine methodological difficulties about this practical and piecemeal approach to the problem. Karl Deutsch makes the point in his defence of the opposite kind of approach to the analysis of the political system:

> We cannot think about particular problems without making assumptions about the general context of the world in which they occur. Usually these assumptions are intuitive and vague. We form some indefinite conception of how states of a particular size and types of government and culture are expected to behave at particular times and places, and we feel surprised when some particular country departs strikingly from these half-formed expectations (Taylor, 1968).

Thus, he argues, indicators can only be derived from a typology of national states, or of political situations, or of mass behaviour patterns; and the only way to arrive at such a typology is on the basis of some theories about the operation of the political system. That, however, is not the same thing as a claim that there must be a comprehensive theoretical system established to cover *all* possible sources of political action as a prior condition for analytical work. Comprehensiveness is the difficulty. It requires the construction of very large aggregates, each bringing together in a single figure a mass of variegated social data. The alternative would contain so many different indicators, of unknown comparative weight, that it would be impossibly complicated to use for any practical purpose. But these jumbo aggregates also raise some acute problems of a conceptual character. A point is discussed by R. A. Dahl in his contribution to *Aggregate Data Analysis* (Taylor, 1968). He concedes that aggregates of the kind used in the *World Handbook of Political and Social Indicators* (Russett *et al.*, 1964) are based on the combination of a variety of indicators whose 'weights assigned may – and generally will – have an arbitrary element', and he goes on to ask whether tests of statistical significance applied to them are 'really valid'. His answer is that validity in this case is determined by the outcome of a species of intellectual shock treatment. To decide whether data of this kind supply important new knowledge 'requires what a distinguished mathematical statistician has called the Inter-Ocular Trauma test of significance: do the results hit you between the eyes?' (op. cit., p. 56).

Now it may well be that this dramatic method will provide some useful insights into the political and social process; several are to be found in the collection of papers brought together in *Aggregate Data Analysis*. But as Goran Ohlin points out in his essay in this collection, some of the assumptions behind the method employed by the political scientists, who wish to proceed at once to the manipulation of very large aggregates in their analysis, are profoundly at variance with those that have been successfully employed hitherto by economists, who have pioneered the use of statistical indicators. As he says,

> economists are inclined to proceed first to a more disaggregated level of the National Accounts, to break down rates of growth, not only to a per capita level but to some 'per unit of input' level, to seek out behavioural aspects like savings-ratios, to combine a cross-sectional approach with that of time series, to be suspicious of data from single years, etc. (ibid., p. 85).

And he concludes:

> Those who seek to relate development variables to non-economic indices seem to proceed in the opposite direction in their use of national income figures: instead of disaggregating they combine them with others, either by reducing a great number of series into few by factor analysis, or by multiple regressions. The first of these techniques, which constructs mysterious patterns or factors of a vague general character out of many well-defined series and does so on purely statistical criteria, strikes me as so utterly alien to an economist's way of looking at things that I cannot say what, if anything, it contributes to our understanding. . . .

Here is the central difficulty. Social scientists concerned with policy formulation must be able to present the relevant data that illuminate the choices to be made in a framework of analysis whose separate items are readily comprehensible to the persons responsible for making political decisions. If the key items presenting the crucial measures of social change are composed of a rag-bag of variegated data, whose combined significance eludes meaningful statement except in terms of the actual process of putting the data together – i.e. in terms of the social scientist's experience that this particular aggregate does provide a representative indicator of certain social processes – the trick is unlikely to work. On the other hand the social scientist outside the field of economics cannot readily manipulate the smaller blocks of disaggregated data, which the economist has learnt to handle with increasing skill, and the reason is the absence of a satisfactory theory about the relationships between the component parts of the system.

The way forward, I would suggest, is to look at the experience of economics before the time when it had developed a usable overall system of measurement in the modern national income accounts. These latter are after all not very old; they were largely developed in the 1930s. Economic indicators did not suddenly come into use at that stage, they had been employed in the making of policy over an extended period before then.

It is indeed striking how the improvement in the quality of the economic data collected and the advances in analysing them during the inter-war period, notably in the United States and Britain, were successful in enlarging the place accorded to economic indicators in the process of policy formulation, even without the backing of a satisfactorily comprehensive theoretical system.

Of course there always were theories to go with the indicators. Economists would not have been themselves if it had been otherwise. My point is only that the individual indicators did not necessarily cease to be useful because the theories that went with them were wrong. Their use, as suggested earlier, was to allow policy-makers to perceive a past trend. It is possible in some cases that such a perception could be worse than perceiving nothing at all; that would be the case if the significance of the trend were grossly misinterpreted in terms of its connections with the rest of the system. But in practice it is by the use of such 'partial indicators' that any science, not merely social science, advances.

Schumpeter (1954) makes an admirable comment on the uses of some well-known pieces of partial economic analysis, based on indicators drawn from a small segment of the economy, in default of a more general theory. He instances the case of the 'pig cycle' – a theory that explained the divergent movement between the price of hogs and the price of corn by observation of the way in which farmers as a body tended to synchronize their decisions to expand or to contract their production. If they were expanding and needed a lot more corn to feed the extra pigs, the price of corn went up while the prices of pigs tended to go down; and vice versa. Of course this kind of analysis based on the observation of the trend in just two price indices has very severe limitations. But, says Schumpeter, such exercises are

> of first order importance; the same reader who is impressed with their shortcomings – much as he would be in reading a description of Columbus' flag-ship – should be also impressed with the fact that an element of the mechanism they describe is undoubtedly present in almost every practical case and, furthermore, with the host of well-defined tasks that they suggest for further work on the same line (p. 1169).

Probably the most considerable systematic effort of this kind undertaken outside the economic sphere is the work done in the US Department of Health, Education, and Welfare (HEW) in the final period of the Johnson Administration. The results were published under the title *Toward a Social Report* at the beginning of 1969 after the change of President.[1] As the title indicates, those responsible were keenly aware of the limitations of this initial exercise. Its chief value probably lies in the insights that it provided into the considerable methodological problems that social scientists still have to face, if the growing body of knowledge at their command is to be brought to bear effectively in the process of government. The social indicators proposed are disaggregated in a way of which Ohlin would approve.

SOME OPERATIONAL DIFFICULTIES

However, even within this more modest conceptual framework the problem of weighting different factors keeps stubbornly asserting itself. For example, the state of the nation's health is measured in approximate terms by means of two indicators: (1) 'expectation of life'; and (2) 'expected bed-disability and institutionalization during life'; and on both counts the evidence suggests that in spite of a continuing rise in the proportion of the national product devoted to medical care, no significant improvement has occurred since the early 1960s. But then, as the Report points out, this measure of the cost-effectiveness of medical care leaves out a factor that the patient himself may regard as extremely important, *viz.* 'the difference in pain and discomfort per day among various diseases'. Pain-killers and sedatives may have made a great difference during this period to the actual experience of each day of 'bed-disability'. There are other problems that enter very deeply into such personal assessments. The social indicators treat the 'dis-utility' of death and of permanent bed-disability as equal; in other words public expenditure that had the effect of reducing either would be treated as being equally beneficial. But is this the view that is in fact taken by the majority of people – in the sense that if they had the freedom to spend money on these two objectives their behaviour would reflect the absence of any preference between one course and the other? The answer is that we do not know. It would also be a laborious exercise to begin to find out.

What emerges very clearly from the discussion of the eight major social objectives that are covered in *Toward a Social Report* is that the lack of information about the attitudes of the consumers of social services is a major weakness in this kind of work. (It is worth saying that it is a weakness that applies equally to the work of economists in the field of cost-benefit analysis.) To construct a small number of sensitive indicators that would reflect in an accurate and convincing fashion trends in criminal behaviour would require some deep investigation of attitudes. The indicators must, if they are to perform their task as an aid to political and social decision, mirror the relative importance that people attach to different kinds of crime. The HEW Report is optimistic about the possibility of a high degree of consensus on this subject: it quotes survey results 'which show that respondents of different classes and occupations tend to agree on the relative heinousness of different significant crimes' and that these correlated very closely with differences in the average length of prison sentences actually given for these crimes. Since the issue of 'law and order' seems to be on the way to becoming a major political question in Western Europe as well as in the United States, clarity on the measures to be applied to the data about the prevalence of various kinds of crime is an urgent matter.

Clearly it will be necessary to keep the composition of the social indicators themselves under constant critical review, in order to ensure that they are closely related to changing social policy objectives. This serves to emphasize their essentially normative character. It is hardly possible to make them morally or politically neutral, since the very notion of a plus and minus on an indicator is influenced by the choice of social goals. If the social indicators are to be kept up to date there will also be a continuing need for a great deal of unweighted data in a disaggregated form. It is to be expected that even if there is broad agreement about the significance of individual measures of social behaviour, the message conveyed by a combination of movements in a given collection of indicators will continue to be the subject of controversy. If, say, sexual crimes went down while drug offences and petty theft were on the increase, questions about the significance of these trends, the relative importance to be attached to the various elements in a social picture, would force themselves upon the public's attention. It is reasonable to expect that the habit of more sophisticated judgement will develop. And one of the by-products of this process, to make politics less volatile and unpredictable, should be a propensity on the part of the general public to view any given segment of the social situation as being the product of a number of different factors not all necessarily pointing in the same direction. This should itself help to make politics a less volatile and unpredictable business.

However, no doubt there will continue to be periodic demands for instant judgement on matters that can in fact be rationally assessed only by means of trends measured over a fairly extended period. Most social indicators are likely to suffer from limitations of this type; fine measurement of small changes over short periods will continue to elude them. It may be that in time certain devices corresponding to 'leading indicators' in the economic field will be found useful as a means of supplying warning signals of a prospective change of trend. Such indicators are not predictive instruments in the full sense; they are merely a collection of readings on a variety of scales that either individually or in combination, have been found from experience to be associated with certain types of social change. But that kind of additional resource for social forecasting is something that lies a long way ahead. The straightforward task of building up the essential data required for the construction of even an elementary array of social indicators will take a considerable time. As Sheldon and Moore say in their introductory essay to *Indicators of Social Change* (1968), 'The temporal order of events, of major structural change, has perhaps suffered from too much observation of concurrent relations and too little observation over longer periods of time. The latter is inherently more difficult, if for no other reason than the fact that observers also move through time, and are not immortal.'

It is worth reiterating that the initial purpose of this exercise is not to create a machine for short-term forecasting, on an analogy with economics, but to put into position monitoring devices that will register, as rapidly as possible, changes that have already taken place. Of course this in itself will increase the efficiency of the apparatus available in the field of public policy for the assessment of future trends. But that has always been the common hope of historians in politics – people who believe that they can discern the probable future better than other politicians because they have a deeper and more accurate knowledge of what has happened in the past. The special contribution of the social indicator to politics lies in providing up-to-date guidance on the data that *should* inform political choices. The 'should' in this context does not mean the introduction of a new moral imperative supplied by social scientists; it merely expresses the fact that given an existing set of moral and political preferences, some of the measurements supplied by the social indicators, and not available without them, are a necessary element in the policy choices to be made.

Although the task of establishing a system of indicators is a long-term one, it is reasonable to expect that the influence of social science on the formulation of the ends of policy will grow substantially in the process. Indeed, there is an example ready to hand of the way in which the process is likely to work, in electoral opinion surveys. The social scientists concerned with the appraisal of voting intentions design questions concerned with aspects of the policies of political parties, which may not be at all those that the leaders of these parties would choose of their own accord to throw into the discussion. In this way the design of an indicator of public opinion may, and sometimes does, alter the terms of the political debate. By probing the deeper springs of popular political sentiment the researchers may have the effect of forcing decisions on issues that the political machines of all the parties in the contest might have preferred to evade or to play down. It is no wonder then that politicians have recently shown increasing nervousness about electoral opinion surveys, and in at least one case (in the West German elections of 1969) have succeeded in imposing a ban on publishing them. There is perhaps a lesson of wider significance to be learned here – that social indicators are too powerful an instrument of public policy to be left to be managed exclusively by governments.

Note

[1] HEW had a Deputy Assistant Secretary for Social Indicators, Mr Mancur Olson, in charge of this work. After the change of administration in 1969 the HEW office was disbanded, but a new office concerned with the same broad range of problems has been established in the White House.

References

GROSS, B. M., *The State of the Nation: Social Systems Accounting.* Tavistock Publications, London, 1966.

KEYNES, J. M., *The General Theory of Employment, Interest, and Money.* Macmillan, London, 1936.

LYONS, G. M., *The Uneasy Partnership: Social Science and the Federal Government in the Twentieth Century.* Russell Sage Foundation, New York, 1969.

RAINWATER, L. and YANCEY, W. L., *The Moynihan Report and the Politics of Controversy.* MIT Press, Cambridge, Mass., 1967.

RIECKEN, H. W., Social Sciences and Social Problems. *Social Science Information* **8**, No. 1, pp. 101–29, 1969.

RUSSETT, B. M., ALKER, H. R., DEUTSCH, K. W., and LASWELL, H. G., *World Handbook of Political and Social Indicators,* Yale University Press, New Haven, Conn., 1965.

SCHUMPETER, J., *History of Economic Analysis,* Oxford University Press, London, 1954.

SHELDON, E. B., and MOORE, W. E. (eds.), *Indicators of Social Change: Concepts and Measurements.* Russell Sage Foundation, New York, 1968.

SHONFIELD, A., *British Economic Policy since the War.* Penguin, Harmondsworth, 1959.

— *Attack on World Poverty*, Random House, New York, 1960.

— *Modern Capitalism.* Oxford University Press, London, 1965.

TAYLOR, C. L. (ed.), *Aggregate Data Analysis.* International Social Science Council, Publication 10, Mouton, Paris, 1968.

US Department of Health, Education, and Welfare, *Toward a Social Report,* US Government Printing Office, Washington, 1969.

Interchapter

In presenting his paper Andrew Shonfield stressed several major points which may be summarized as follows.

To a greater degree than any other social scientists, economists have been brought fully into the policy-making process, being involved not only in discussing the *means* of achieving certain ends, but in discussing the *ends* themselves. One reason for this is that economics had developed a comprehensive system of explanation of the relationship between the various parts of the economy, so, in principle, an economist can explain how an action in one sector of the economy may affect another sector.

However, economists do not always produce the same answers to a given problem, nor, indeed, are these answers inevitably correct. What is important is that economic criteria and the way the economic system works are matters of broad agreement between economists at any one time. These matters of broad agreement provide the theoretical underpinning to the work of the different economists.

Even before this comprehensive explanation of the economic system was developed, economists worked on establishing key indicators of economic change, which can be understood and used by policy-makers.

The other social sciences have not, as yet, developed a comprehensive explanatory system of society, nor does it appear likely that they will in the near future. Rather than wait until this possibly utopian objective has been achieved, they should start work now towards the development of indicators of social change.

There are however many dangers in thinking that social indicators can be used in a similar way to economic indicators. Without a theoretical explanation of society, you cannot use indicators of the large aggregate type that economists manipulate. But if we disaggregate our data, then not only do we lack leading indicators that can be used as predictors, but we are faced with the problems of weighting several small disparate indicators, for if they are to be usable, we must devise some means of making them comparable.

One reason why economics and psychology are used more, especially in the USA, is that they offer policy-makers usable information. If the other social scientists wish to follow this example, and convert social data into material conveniently available for the policy-maker, then they must tackle the problems of multiple choice, and relative importance.

Shonfield cited the case of the siting of London's third airport as an example of the importance of understanding the problems of multiple choice and relative importance. The Roskill Commission was attempting to bring together all the evidence presented by experts concerning such things as the social and psychological effects of noise, the various costs that would accrue due to the relative distance from London of the various sites, the cost of disrupting country life, and similar factors. But, as was apparent, no amount of 'evidence' from 'experts' can replace the need for value judgements of the relative importance of conflicting points of view.[1] Values were frequently incommensurable, and social science cannot, in the form of indicators or any other techniques, provide a substitute. Thus it is vital that the social scientists be involved in several stages of the policy-making process, rather than function simply as technicians who supply data, on which decisions are made automatically. Economists have achieved this status; the other social scientists have yet to do so.

This exercise in measuring economic and social costs and benefits also raises the question of how we select the elements to include in the equation, and how they are to be measured; how are the arguments presented by an articulate, well-organized pressure group to be weighted against the opinions of less articulate individuals? These are just a few examples of the many problems to be solved before administrators can use social accounting as they now use economic indicators.

While members of the Conference saw the development of the use of social indicators as an exciting challenge to social scientists, they were wary of modelling them too closely on present economic indicators. For example, the relative success by economists in using indicators is based on a deft use of the *ceteris paribus* principle. In theoretical models of the economy, certain variables can be held constant, while the effect on others is studied; but holding the variables constant in this manner is not appropriate in the study of human society.

The danger of a system of social indicators is that they will be regarded as conclusive and exhaustive, and policy-makers will be bound by them. This happened with economic indicators, and we are now trying to break away from it. Some economic indicators have become so entrenched in our way of thinking that we are in danger of losing the ability to change with changing situations. Rather than a system of interrelated indicators, we need *many* indicators that can reflect the relative importance that different individuals may attach to them, and can be regarded as flexible.

If policy-makers only encourage the development of social indicators in those areas where they are politically feasible, as was the case with *Toward a Social Report*, published by the US Department of Health, Education, and Welfare (HEW), then they do not hold out a very exciting challenge. But if the work in developing social indicators, particularly social psychological indicators, can awaken and broaden the concerns of policy-makers, if it can encourage 'imagination stretching', then it will be more worth while. Some current work being carried out in the US, and reported in the recent volume by Moore & Sheldon (1968), reflects a conscious effort to counterbalance the rather simplistic use of politically acceptable indicators in the HEW Report, by moving towards theoretically derived social indicators. These can suggest to policy-makers alternative objectives that they may not previously have considered.

A study of attitudes to housing was given as an example of how social psychological indicators can be used to broaden the perspective of the policy sector. This particular study showed that while the feelings of well-being and participation among the white sector of the lower-income groups increased with improved housing conditions, among the black community an increase in the standards of housing increased feelings of alienation. Hence, depth indicators which probe the variables intervening between action and response appear to be necessary for meaningful policy-making. Indicators constructed on a gross level (e.g. indicators of housing standards that ignore the characteristics of the inhabitants) run the risk of providing erroneous information. We constantly need new indicators – this entails the close scrutiny of critical social processes. Large natural experiments present an ideal opportunity for assessing the kind of indicators that are most useful. The change from right-hand to left-hand driving in Sweden gave a unique chance of reassessing the assumptions about traffic problems, the differing attitudes and perceptions of the population, not only to traffic, but also the process of rapid change. Similarly, the change to decimal currency in Britain presents another opportunity for such studies.

One participant saw the actual achievement of social indicators as less important than the renewed emphasis on theoretical development that the attempt to derive social indicators would encourage. The development of theoretically derived social indicators presents the real challenge to both social scientists and policy-makers.

Returning to the issue of economics as an example of the other disciplines in relating to policy-makers, the danger of regarding economics as different, for whatever reasons, was pointed out. For too long it has been assumed that the economic sector is independent from the rest of society and can be administered and manipulated without taking account of the repercussions in the wider realms of society. Alongside the emergence of policy-oriented social scientists and the developments of interdisciplinary subjects such as policy science, has grown an awareness of the need to conceptualize larger, more comprehensive systems of society, interrelating social, economic, and political subsystems.

Note

[1] When the Roskill Commission reported in January 1971, although they made a choice of where the airport should be sited, based on their estimates of social and economic costs, they thought the ultimate decision of weighting the various elements was a political one, and should be made by the politicians.

Part 2

Aspects of Social Science Policy

5 The need for and provision of social science manpower[1]

Dietrich Goldschmidt

Policies for the social sciences, irrespective of their cultural settings, and of the degree of central control involved, must deal with issues such as the provision and allocation of scarce resources (both money and manpower) and the creation and maintenance of institutional bases within which teaching, research, and associated activities in the social sciences can be initiated and developed. The next three chapters deal with aspects of this problem, approached both from a general level and from the perspective of a particular cultural context.

Manpower planning is a topic that in recent years has generated much discussion but little comprehension. Even in highly specified professional fields such as the natural sciences and engineering, attempts to match manpower production, principally from the higher education sector, with manpower demand as set out by the employment sector, both public and private, have rarely ended in success. Further, the impact of trained personnel in organizations themselves has seldom been taken into account, i.e. the rate of growth in demand has frequently been projected as linear rather than as changing continually over time.

If such difficulties are experienced in projecting demand in the comparatively well-defined and specific professions, the problems in estimating for less determinate occupations, such as the social sciences, become all too apparent. Outside occasional surveys within particular countries, little in the way of statistical information of the present state and growth of manpower resources in the social sciences is available. Even less is known of the impact of personnel trained in the social sciences on various employment sectors.

In this chapter, Dietrich Goldschmidt outlines some of the problems encountered in manpower studies, illustrating his account with examples from the German situation. He draws attention to the difficulties in defining the 'trained social scientist' and to the need to mount dynamic studies to investigate the mobility of trained personnel and their impact as an innovative force in society. No trained political scientists existed in Germany before 1945, hence it has been possible to initiate pilot studies on the absorption of new political science graduates into professional life. In conclusion, Goldschmidt points to the importance of examining the higher education system as the major source of social science manpower and makes some suggestions for widening the scope of the disciplines within this system.

Director of the Institute for Educational Research in the Max-Planck-Gesellschaft in Berlin, Dietrich Goldschmidt is a sociologist whose current work deals with problems of higher and secondary education. Publications include (with M. Jenne) Educational Sociology in the Federal Republic of Germany (1969); *Educational Planning and Educational Research* (Festschrift for Otto Brenner, 1968).

For two reasons it is somewhat difficult to discuss the structural requirements for social science manpower and trace the lines of professional training and status in the field. On one hand several extensive and fairly detailed reports have been published in the past few years covering the present situation in the social sciences with respect to their objectives and manpower problems (BASS Survey, 1969; Crawford, 1970; NSF Report, 1969; OECD, 1966; Sinclair, 1968–70; UNESCO, 1968). On the other hand there has not been sufficient effort to clarify the situation of the social sciences by comparing national statistics. It still remains to evaluate this material systematically. In particular, new categories and statistical tools have to be used in order to trace those various trends in the scientific field which are labelled as 'social' ones.

DEFINITION OF SOCIAL SCIENCES AND OF SOCIAL SCIENCE MANPOWER

> The term 'social sciences' is used here to cover the complex of disciplines concerned with the behaviour of man in society and of social institutions. These include sociology, psychology, economics, political science, demography, social anthropology, the social aspects of legal, historical, and geographical studies. Each of these disciplines is distinct in specialization and character, and each has its intellectual and methodological approach to problems. All however make use of mathematical and statistical tools, and different types of model-building (OECD, 1966, p. 21).

That the social sciences operate by 'scientific methods' comparable to those that are applied in the natural sciences is the conception of all its members as far as their scientific status is concerned. Research is conducted according to principles of observation that claim objectivity on the basis of interpersonal agreement on the validity of the methods. Not unlike the natural sciences, the social sciences are kept free of value judgements when facts are collected. However, one should keep in mind that the definition of a problem in terms of social research always reflects value judgements, vested interests, and political decisions. The results therefore can be, and very often are, brought to bear on the formulation of social policy. That is why social sciences usually serve politics in the broadest sense of the term and prepare the way for political decisions.

Social scientists, seen in this context, may be described as 'Servants of Power' according to the provocative title of Baritz's book (1960). In general they are engaged in very different institutions of a society; they may be teachers, administrators, journalists, or researchers. The latter will be the object of our reflections here, as they constitute the scientific spearhead of the whole group. However, there are certain difficulties in identifying researchers on the basis of the given statistics. In this connection Cherns and Sinclair (1968) are justified in contending that a BA or an equivalent degree in social science does not generally qualify a college graduate as a 'researcher'. However, those who remain at the university in order to work for an advanced degree in social sciences – for a PhD in particular – are very likely to devote part of their time to research.[2] Furthermore, it can be assumed that those who stay at the university after having been awarded the doctoral degree will generally continue their research work. Should they however leave the university at this point, it is practically impossible to determine whether and to what extent they carry on working in the field of research or instead take up jobs as teachers, administrators, journalists, and so on. As the training of social scientists, including that of doctoral candidates, is less specific than that of natural scientists, they are more likely to vary their occupation from time to time. They have a broad range of job opportunities as 'generalists' within different organizational settings. In the case of those working in research outside the universities it is difficult to determine to what extent their inquiries are 'pure research' or just means for carrying out their jobs as administrators or teachers, for instance. How, for example, does one categorize surveys conducted for a particular administration? Where does the observation of classroom interaction and the testing of new teaching methods fit in?

Social science research gains in importance in proportion to the extent to which its findings are applied in practice. The social sciences function as an ever greater innovative force in society as their representatives move to and fro between research and action, between theory and practice. Something that restricts and possibly even abolishes a social scientist's freedom of movement between these two fields is the tendency to rank the different activities in accordance with the view of academic work as indicator of qualification and prestige. In other professions, such as teaching, outmoded qualification barriers are by now breaking down or being reduced to their functionally necessary core. Under such circumstances it would be unjustifiable in terms of social policy to create a distinction between the social researcher, other social scientists, and social workers. The interplay of social problems and theoretical concepts and their two-way enrichment becomes seriously endangered when social science researchers are separated from the rest of their professional community. As a 'crucial problem in all countries', the OECD Report stresses the relations between research, training, and university structures (OECD, 1966, p. 67). While qualified research should be based on interdisciplinary collaboration, it says, the traditional framework of universities usually does not allow such a synthesis. The system of short-term research contracts for university members is the factor primarily responsible for the lack of continuity and cumulation in social research. Besides, the teaching load on academic social scientists is reported to have become a serious obstacle to the conduct of research in many universities, entailing a separation between teaching departments and university research institutes (OECD, 1966, p. 68).

INSTITUTIONALIZATION OF THE SOCIAL SCIENCES

The different individual disciplines that constitute the social sciences are part of the universities' teaching programme in all countries here considered: Belgium, the Federal Republic of Germany, France, Great Britain, Italy, and the USA. Usually the scientists' main concern is to develop the disciplines distinct from one another, sometimes even in conflict with one another. However, multi- or interdisciplinary research has its only chance to succeed when the social sciences are called upon to aid in solving social problems of immediate relevance. Ordinarily the objectives, means, and extensions of interdisciplinary research do not fit into the departmental structure of universities, which requires that extra-university institutes be established. There are, in fact, seven different kinds of research establishments to be discerned:

1. university departments or institutes;
2. independent research institutes with, for the most part, non-commissioned, fixed budgets;
3. independent research institutes working on publicly commissioned products;
4. research institutes that are direct subsidiaries of government or similar agencies;
5. sections of government departments for administrative research;
6. private institutes operating on a commerical basis;
7. industrial departments for company research and business and labour associations.

These various forms of research organization do not fit the traditional distinction between basic and applied research. Interdisciplinary research is becoming more and more important, creating, of course, its own theoretical and methodological problems. What has a strong bearing on their solution is the fact that these various forms of research organization determine to a certain extent the way a project is approached and carried out and how its findings are publicized. The more problem-orientated a research programme is, the more directly it can influence political decisions; the more dependent research is, the more it serves one-sided interests and concerns (Scheuch, 1969, 1970). Independence of research may provide contributions to social justice and to democratic action within a given society. This is to a very high degree 'political' research serving the 'national interest'. This statement may meet with disagreement; most of the reports at hand seem to be haunted, as it were, by the vision of the nonpartisan, coolly disinterested scholar who only wants to let his research results speak for themselves. One need not be a Marxist to demonstrate that such contentions serve to obscure vested interests or reflect a degree of naïveté that is almost unpardonable for a social scientist (cf. the work of C. Wright Mills or Baritz's *Servants of Power*, 1960). The manifest political function of social science research is most clearly demonstrated in the great number of advisory bodies connected with ministries and other government agencies throughout the world. If we look at the German Federal Republic, there were about 70 such advisory bodies reported in October 1966 (Dreitzel, 1966). Though they do not make political decisions, their recommendations weigh strongly in the decision-making process, and to this extent they have a definite political function (Friedrich, 1970).

CORRESPONDENCE BETWEEN MANPOWER NEEDS AND THE PROVISION OF MANPOWER IN THE SOCIAL SCIENCES

It is by now almost common knowledge that there exists a rapidly growing need for social science research throughout the world (NSF Report, 1969). The goals of research vary from country to country, depending on the socioeconomic and political structure of each state. As to the extent of their research, the social sciences still lag far behind the natural sciences,[3] but with reference to the student population the field of social sciences is constantly growing. In Japan, for example, the number of undergraduate social sciences students has even outpaced those in the natural sciences and technology. The reasons for such a trend in the academic field are quite manifold, being motivationally, institutionally, or politically determined. In any case the social sciences are relatively freely accessible, so that the field can absorb all those students who are excluded from other academic courses because of insufficient capacity (for instance, science and technology in Japan, medicine in the German Federal Republic).

Growing numbers of students lead to a corresponding increase in the number of graduates. That is why the present situation of the labour market for social scientists can be described as one in which graduates of 'new' subjects like sociology or political science try to increase their job opportunities by working for a doctoral degree (König, 1966; Rudd and Hatch, 1968). They offer qualifications not demanded by any official employer, and find jobs in an unusual, not yet institutionalized way. The ordinary model of the functioning of the labour market does not suit this case. The contradistinction of 'need' to 'provision' of manpower leads one to believe that the system of higher education is automatically providing the necessary kinds and numbers of qualified scientists. In reality, this pattern can only be applied to neatly structured careers within the traditional professional systems. In a relatively new academic field, such as that of the social sciences, the supply of trained personnel is pushing into the market. Here the supply is creating the demand; no need as such necessarily assures the provision of social scientists. Given the opportunity to go about their inquiries within existing or new research institutions and thereby to function as innovators, these research workers are 'absorbed' by the institutions employing them without this system having previously indicated more than, at best, a diffuse need for their services.

To elucidate the process of absorption, I should like to describe the results of a pilot study on 'political scientists in professional life', which was conducted recently by the Institute for Educational Research in the Max-Planck-Gesellschaft, Berlin.[4] The study indicated that 32 per cent of all political scientists interviewed held jobs that they themselves had been able to define, i.e. that had not existed before. Together with the 12 per cent who took up jobs already structured by predecessors of the same qualifications, this means that 44 per cent of all persons interviewed were engaged in an occupation that corresponded roughly to the professional training they had received. An equally large percentage, however, was holding positions which hitherto had been occupied either by nongraduates or by people trained in other academic fields (15 per cent without any academic qualification; 29 per cent university graduates in other fields). Measuring the fluctuation in these relatively well-entrenched positions, one could find that, though temporarily filled by political scientists, they usually reverted back to people whose qualifications resembled those of the original job-holders. When they graduate, German political scientists are not equipped with any great degree of detailed knowledge in special fields of practical relevance. Their 'strength' lies in their very general, unspecialized training, which enables them to give structure to jobs not yet tightly circumscribed but involving a wide range of activities.

The Institute for Educational Research (Institut für Bildungsforschung, Berlin) will carry on with its research into the absorption of highly qualified manpower in the employment system in order to provide a better insight into the process of ongoing innovation and, if possible, come to some more general conclusions.

PROVISION OF SOCIAL SCIENCE MANPOWER

At colleges and universities, social science studies are presented in three ways, thus providing for three types of graduates or postgraduates trained in social sciences:

1. A discipline in the field of the social sciences constitutes a major subject for college students who, upon graduation with a Bachelor's or equivalent degree, want to enter professional life as social workers, solicitors, teachers, accountants, administrators, etc. or to proceed into postgraduate studies (UGC Report, 1968, pp. 18, 19, 26, 27; Abbott, 1969).
2. Social science disciplines provide the main focus of postgraduate studies for oncoming social researchers.
3. Social science disciplines represent supplementary subjects for non-majors: undergraduate as well as graduate students who are training for ordinary professions – such as law, medicine, engineering, journalism, public administration, etc. (NSF Report, 1969, p. 21).

At this point a further differentiation can be made. Social science graduates may either qualify themselves to carry out practical research work in various public institutions or they may devote themselves to hermeneutical reflection and critical social theory. The former, as they go into their jobs, will be integrated into a part of the general social system that can be improved or modernized only when organizational needs require. However, it is unlikely that an individual doing his research work for such an institution could promote much profound internal change by himself. If this is true, any social researcher doing his work in this kind of framework functions as a system-stabilizing force, regardless of the fact that he sees himself as someone who is contributing to social innovation.

The other group of graduate students tends to develop a more unyielding and uncompromising view of present societies; therefore its members are very likely to work with relatively independent research institutes, which are oriented towards basic research or basic issues, if they do not stay at the university for research or teaching purposes (cf. the situation of the sociologists in the Federal Republic of Germany: Schlottmann, 1968). The utilization of social sciences in professions of traditional standing must lead to a certain scientific reorientation. To make use of the social sciences cannot simply mean to fit them into the existing curricula; what is necessary is the 'sensitizing' of experts to the social consequences of their professional behaviour. Besides, they should learn to think in terms of sociological correlations and social interaction, so that they can act in a responsible and humane way when they are confronted with the problems of their professions.[5]

Taking all the trends together, the social sciences have become today's foremost science of orientation. In some countries and in certain disciplines, however, this insight has not yet changed reality. Students, in their protest movements, are pressing more than anyone else for scientific rethinking. But the task of integrating the social sciences into other disciplines needs more than this; it also requires the interest and goodwill of scholars and scientists in order that they may permeate each other's fields. Interdisciplinary groups of teachers and students working on projects that have emerged out of practical problems, such as town planning or air pollution, may mean a great step towards the integration of the social sciences.

Such considerations lead to the conclusion that – in addition to the three above-mentioned ways of training social scientists – specific supplementary courses or seminars should be developed in which the didactics of the social sciences, their theory and methods in relation to the demands of these disciplines and to those of the students, would be worked out in colleges and universities. By this the university teacher might qualify himself as a specific type of social scientist. His particular task would be to give special attention to the possible contribution of social sciences to social development; to interaction between theory and practice; to demands on the social sciences by society; and to the aims and expectations of students. In practical terms, this would also require that teacher and student develop courses of study with special consideration in the curricula for task-oriented interdisciplinary studies. However, there is a possible pitfall in this further specialization: if, for the sake of integrating the social sciences, a special position is created within the existing structure of jobs, no fundamental change may occur with regard to co-operation between the already established positions. To achieve this, one needs a permanent and perhaps institutionalized alternation between research and teaching, practical social work and abstract theorizing. If it is true that social sciences have to 'experience' the whole of reality, its various branches cannot simply reduce their sensory complexity to 'one-way streets' of either observation or action. If social science researchers wanted to see themselves established as a profession for the purpose of securing and preserving status, such as doctors and lawyers have established, then they would be behaving contrary to their profession's political mandate, which is to serve the emancipation of the people and the democratization of society.

Notes

[1] The author is indebted to Miss Sibylle Funk, who kindly prepared this manuscript for publication.

[2] Cf. Work of University Teachers in Term and Vacation, according to the 'Robbins Report' (OECD, 1966, p. 94).

[3] Cf. Belgian Figures on 'Manpower on Scientific Activities: Social Sciences compared with Natural Sciences' (OECD, 1966, p. 95).

[4] Hartung, Nuthmann, and Winterhager, 1970. It should be kept in mind that the research was concerned with a relatively small population. It was based on questionnaires that were put to 708 persons who graduated in political science in the years 1951 to 1968 at the Free University of Berlin, the only German institution to offer a diploma in political science.

[5] Teachers, for example, should not only learn to conceive their role within the social context of school-administration, parents, and pupils, but also change the way of interpreting their subjects. In the Federal Republic of Germany such a process of scientific reorientation has just started at the teacher-training colleges as well as in certain branches of the humanities such as German philology.

References

ABBOTT, J., Employment of Sociology and Anthropology Graduates, 1966–67: A Report of Research Surveys. British Sociological Association, London, 1969.

BARITZ, L., *Servants of Power: A History of Social Science in American Industry*. Wesleyan University Press, Middletown, Conn., 1960.

Behavioral and Social Sciences Survey Committee (BASS), *The Behavioral and Social Sciences: Outlook and Needs*. Prentice-Hall, Englewood Cliffs, N.J., 1969.

CHERNS, A. B., and SINCLAIR, R., Social Science Policy. Paper presented at Loughborough Conference on Social Science Policy, 1968; revised as a working paper for the International Conference, Paris, 1970.

CRAWFORD, E. T., The Sociology of the Social Sciences: An International Bibliography. *Social Science Information* **9**, 1, 1970.

DREITZEL, D., Die Bundesregierung und ihre Wissenschaftler. *Atomzeitalter* **10**, pp. 295–9, 1966.

FRIEDRICH, H., *Staatliche Verwaltung und Wissenschaft: Die wissenschaftliche Beratung der Politik aus der Sicht der Ministerialbürokratie*. Europäische Verlagsanstalt, Frankfurt am M., 1970.

GOLDSCHMIDT, D., *Educational Planning and Educational Research*, 1968.

GOLDSCHMIDT, D., and JENNE, M., Educational Sociology in the Federal Republic of Germany. *Social Science Information* **8**, 4, pp. 19–29, 1969.

HARTUNG, D., NUTHMANN, R., and WINTERHAGER, W. D., *Politologen im Beruf: Zur Aufnahme und Durchsetzung neuer Qualifikationen im Beschäftigungssystem*. Klett, Stuttgart, 1970.

KÖNIG, R., Das Lehren der Soziologie in entwickelten und unterentwickelten Ländern. *Kölner Zeitschrift für Soziologie und Sozialpsychologie* **18**, 4, pp. 638–70, 1966.

National Science Foundation, *Knowledge into Action: Improving the Nation's Use of the Social Sciences*. NSB 69–3, US Government Printing Office, Washington, 1969.

OECD, The Social Sciences and the Policies of Governments. Paris, 1966.

RUDD, E., and HATCH, S., *Graduate Study and After*. London, Weidenfeld and Nicolson, 1968.

SCHEUCH, E. K., Sozialforschung in Europa und Politik. *VWF Mitteilungen*, No. 3, 1969; No. 1, 1970.

SCHLOTTMANN, U., Soziologen im Beruf: Zur beruflichen Situation der Absolventen eines soziologischen Studiums in Deutschland: erster Bericht über eine Untersuchung. *Kölner Zeitschrift für Soziologie und Sozialpsychologie* **20**, No. 3, 1968.

SINCLAIR, R., Bibliography of Social Science Policy. Vols 1, 2, 3. Centre for Utilization of Social Science Research, Loughborough University of Technology, 1968–70.

UNESCO, *The Social Sciencés: Problems and Orientations. Selected Studies*. Mouton, Paris, 1968.

University Grants Committee, *First Employment of University Graduates, 1966–67*. HMSO, London, 1968.

Interchapter

Dietrich Goldschmidt's paper initiated a debate on strategies for research and manpower support and the results of some of these as currently practised; and on the general issues of education and training.

On the first topic, Jeremy Mitchell, Secretary of the British Social Science Research Council (SSRC), outlined the position that existed within the UK. There is a consensus both from within the disciplines and from natural scientists and technologists that social science should be expanded; yet the amount of expansion was small. Preliminary studies identify three major constraints to growth, namely money, manpower, and organization. Only 2·6 per cent of the budget for the UK research councils goes to the social sciences; yet, even on this low scale, distribution of resources poses consistent difficulties and a good proportion of research proposals are rejected. To tackle manpower scarcities, several new training programmes have been established and over 50 per cent of the SSRC's budget goes on postgraduate training. The effects of these programmes are difficult to evaluate precisely but Mr Mitchell was pessimistic of their overall effects. Social science in the UK pays too little attention to research methods and training and also lacks a clearly defined research tradition (unlike the natural sciences) which provides criteria to judge what is good research and what is not. As far as organization is concerned, social science research units in universities lack continuity, and similar institutional constraints cause difficulties outside university structures. Hence, people of high quality have little opportunity to devote the necessary time to research and in addition there is some opposition to organized team research. Thus the provision of extended support for workers of proven capabilities and the encouragement of research teams are important factors in any overall research strategy.

Albert Cherns saw much of the situation Mitchell had depicted as all too familiar, but added three points. First, one must consider the importance of the substantive areas and thus take account of the non-homogeneity of the social sciences. Differences exist even within disciplines and the presence of such distinct traditions acts as the focus for many discussions and disputes. The development of strategies embracing all areas indiscriminately is therefore a questionable policy. Second, any movement towards rapid expansion will mean (and has meant) manpower dilution; in particular, research training is often carried out by people lacking experience in research. Finally, many pockets of traditional experience in research lie outside universities in institutes. This leads to many difficulties, not the least of which is the problem of associating such structures with patterns of institutional support.

Taking up some of the points of Mitchell and Cherns, Andrew Shonfield considered that although what they had said was undoubtedly significant the importance of cultural traditions seemed to have been overlooked. Taking the example of teamwork – is there in particular countries (or even in particular disciplines or areas) a resistance to this style of working? In economics in the US one appears to follow a tradition of looking for a team, even in circumstances where one man might possibly operate more efficiently; this contrasts sharply with patterns in the UK. On the more general topic of the social sciences in Britain, Shonfield agreed with Albert Cherns regarding manpower dilution. The expansion of social sciences in the universities has almost completely taken up the top talent available. Some men have been rushed into professorial chairs at a very early stage, often to the detriment of their research. Hence, expansion has a cost that is frequently forgotten in the formation and implementation of plans for growth.

However, if the British situation did not lack internal critics, neither did it lack external support from some of the European participants in the discussion, and Bertrand de Jouvenel took Jeremy Mitchell to task for 'the Britishness' of his approach. He had a long acquaintance with the development of the social sciences, both in the UK and in Europe, and during this period Britain had frequently taken the lead with regard to both institution-building and the development of lines of research. What better example to point to than the continued work of an organization such as Political and Economic Planning (PEP), while as an instance of new lines of research there immediately sprang to his mind the studies involved in the pioneering of new towns.

Further contributions from participants confirmed that the British situation looked somewhat less gloomy to outside observers, although Henning Friis considered that while he saw nothing frightening about developments in the UK, what really disturbed him was the situation internationally. He linked this with the need for an interdisciplinary approach and with recent efforts in Denmark to draft a Bachelor's course to cover the whole of the social sciences. This is one innovation within Scandinavia that has been generally accepted by the universities.

On broader issues of education and training, Cherns wondered whether higher degrees, as typified by the PhD structure in the UK and the US, did not imply a contradiction. While the award of the PhD is regarded as a licence to undertake research, to acquire it an individual is forced to perform work on his own. One result of this is that the PhD is an inadequate, or worse than inadequate, preparation for collaborative research. Some institutions are trying to devise systems whereby the PhD can be awarded for shared work, but this becomes more difficult as one moves to domain-based research. Possibly we need to differentiate between the PhD as evidence of ability to provide original thought and as a certificate of research training. The PhD however is not the sole culprit here – it is essentially an indicator of the difficulties of organizing work on an interdisciplinary or problem-oriented base within university structures.

Cherns's claim that universities frequently have an inhibiting rather than a broadening effect was taken up by Orville Brim, who pointed to the importance of the professional schools (e.g. medicine, law, etc.) in America. It is here that future policy-makers are to be found rather than in social science departments, which tend to produce what the policy-makers see as introverted products: graduates who can criticize and strike down established institutions, but who offer nothing in their place. This criticism however did not include economists, since although they (like sociologists and political scientists) strike at existing institutions, they offer alternative theories to replace those they attack. In short, they possessed a utilizable expertise and this makes both economists and their work more readily applicable to policy.

Other speakers, notably Professors Thorsrud and Carvalho, expressed a concern with the numbers of social science graduates being produced in their respective countries compared to the number of job opportunities available. But Professor Jolles doubted that this implied an oversupply of graduates; only about half of the students studying social science do so with particular professional futures in mind. In his experience, many of them just want a general academic education. Thus, in Holland, many social science graduates move into administration: the labour movement; management; and government. Like the products of the US professional schools mentioned by Orville Brim, they act as links between academic social science and the polity; hence, it is unnecessary to worry that graduates do not have clearcut career lines before them.

Yet to Einar Thorsrud the Scandinavian situation distinctly differs from that of Holland. In Norway, for example, few social science students enter the professional positions described by Jolles; rather, they tend to remain within the university system. Furthermore, those social scientists who do move into professional areas are so completely socialized in their new environment that they either forget or discard all their social science.

In summing up, Professor Goldschmidt warned against treating these topics on too general a level. The social sciences cover many disciplines and the need for trained manpower differs from country to country and from discipline to discipline. What we require are national studies disaggregated by discipline. For example, in Germany, the education of economists has a long tradition and there are recognized economic professions. However, there were no political scientists and few sociologists until 1945 and any analysis will have to take into account the time of establishment of a particular discipline. Another difficulty is that the ambitions of many social science students, namely to solve social problems, differ from those of the professors whose interests lie in academic social research. In Germany the steady increase in the numbers of students of sociology means a widening gap between their motivation and that of their professors. Thus, although our present institutions adequately foster disciplinary development, the need is for institutions for interdisciplinary and problem-oriented research. The requirement for a combination of theory and action is changing some of the European universities from elite organizations to broader structures. Linking them with action means more research training aimed particularly at remedying backwardness of specific sectors. The need to tackle concrete problems, for research in neglected areas and for the development of research training, cannot be considered separately; together they point to an explicit policy for social science manpower.

6 Types of output mix of research organizations and their complementarity

Eric Trist

A major factor governing the legitimation and successful advancement of both teaching and research activities in the social sciences is their accommodation within a defined institutional base. In discussing developments and innovations in both the natural and social sciences, it has become almost commonplace to consider the higher education system as the most 'appropriate' institutional location for research activities. However, as institutional forms proliferate to accommodate activities that are increasing in number and diversifying in content, it becomes necessary sometimes to reject this location as too narrow and stultifying.

Attacking the problems of the organization of research on a general, cross-cultural level, Eric Trist, in a detailed and comprehensive chapter, argues that social research and policy are becoming increasingly interrelated and that this is affecting the nature and character of research organizations. Social research he considers to be an activity becoming increasingly more 'domain'-based, understood only from the viewpoint of systems theory, an approach that attempts to integrate rather than fragment the disciplines. At the same time policy has become anticipatory rather than corrective, seeking to reduce uncertainty through future orientation, and to account for interdependence of elements through comprehensiveness. Such changes have together led to the emergence of new forms of scientific activity, in particular those that can be included in the category of problem-oriented social research.

These different types of activity are best accommodated in different types of organization and in the second part of his chapter Trist develops at length typologies of research organization. He examines how institutional location may control organizational activities, and how such organizations may need to relate to other institutions and sectors. He also considers the structure of social research organizations, particularly how this relates to the 'critical mass' necessary for the organization to operate effectively. The arguments are illustrated with examples drawn from Trist's comprehensive, internationally based knowledge of social research institutes and organizations. His basic aim is to develop a general model of institutional forms through which certain underlying structural conditions and key relationships can be identified. Within such a framework the idiomatic nature of certain organizational forms is not disputed.

At present Professor in the Management Science Center at the Wharton School of Finance and Commerce, University of Pennsylvania, Eric Trist was formerly Chairman of the Committee of Management of the Tavistock Institute, London (1958–66), and Professor of Organizational Behavior at the University of California (1967–9). His major interest has been in examining the interrelations of the technical, economic, and social aspects of organizations within a systems framework. Publications include *Explorations in Group Relations* (with C. Sofer, 1959), *Organizational Choice* (with G. Higgin *et al.*, 1963) and 'Organization and Financing of Social Science Research' (in *The Main Trends of Research in the Social and Human Sciences*, 1970).

INTRODUCTION

For many purposes, including the present, the structure of organizations is most suitably analysed and appraised in terms of what they do, the tasks that they are created to perform. We shall therefore consider the scientific activities of organizations concerned with research in any of the disciplines or interdisciplines of the social sciences as constituting an *output mix*. We shall attempt to identify the basic forms that these mixes take in different contexts and the combinations to which they can give rise.

There are many ways of classifying research and other organizations. One, congruent with that presented here, is the scheme proposed by Cherns (1970) for a distinct but related purpose. Both schemes aim to further the development of a theory of application for the social sciences, the need for which has recently been emphasized by Brim (1970). Now that societies, developed and developing, are attempting to utilize the social sciences on a scale and in ways not earlier contemplated – though still with questionable success – the need to make headway with a theory of application has become a matter of some urgency. Even the rudiments scarcely yet exist. Moreover, much confusion has been caused by supposing that the process of applying the social sciences must somehow be identical with that of applying the natural sciences. A fundamental difference exists in a number of the major areas of inquiry which has far-reaching implications for the way the research effort is organized. The difference consists in this: access to some, though not all, of the many kinds of data required (but these data are among the most important) has to be secured in their natural setting – that is, in society rather than in the laboratory – and as these data are people, their permission has to be asked before they will make themselves available.

Before examining this and other questions we must notice another cardinal fact: certain critical changes have been taking place in the concepts of what science is about and in the matters with which public policy concerns itself. Since the Second World War a growing number of countries have come to accept both science policies and policy sciences – bringing to the fore a type of scientific activity best regarded as distinct from either basic or applied research. We shall refer to this as *domain based*. Domain-based research has very special importance for the social sciences as a means of advancing the frontiers of knowledge, as well as of contributing to human betterment. Unless this is understood the function of a major class of research organizations, which we have called the *special* institutes, will be misperceived.

Domain-based research is inherently interdisciplinary, since a major societal problem has multiple aspects. Beyond endeavour which is collaborative it requires group creativeness. To achieve this at a higher level than is usually attained poses difficult problems for scientists nurtured in a tradition of individualism. Changes in the values of scientists and in the culture of scientific organizations are called for. These matters will be touched on in our concluding section. Their importance may be more readily apparent once an analysis in some depth has been made of the main organizational forms in the fundamental, domain-based, and applied areas of research. The complementarity of output mixes will be stated in systems terms. The characteristics of each will be related to the distinctive competence required for the function performed.

CHANGES IN SCIENCE AND POLICY AND THEIR INTERRELATIONS

New Concepts of Science

Three changes have occurred that have made science more 'human' than it seemed several decades ago. These are the abandonment of the belief in total explanation, the abandonment of reductionism, and the appearance of an integrative, in addition to an analytic, strategy.

The scientific world view, which prevailed in the nineteenth century, and which still haunts the popular image of science, was not reconcilable with human values. It was based on a model of mechanism, atomism, and determinism, and so scarcely depicted a world that men could live in. The coming of the relativity and uncertainty principles upset this view in the physical sciences. The more sophisticated concepts that have followed have removed the omniscience from science. The scientist can no longer lay claim to the whole truth – to total explanation (Polanyi, 1967). There are other forms of understanding. This situation had to exist before scientists, professionals, administrators, and politicians could collaborate in relations of mutual respect (Price, 1965). It is a necessary condition for a positive science policy, which depends on bringing together these four 'estates'.

Next, the advent of open system and information theory in biology upset the principle of reductionism. Other options are now available to explain the negentropy of the 'living'. Moreover, these advances in biology are assisting the social sciences in finding their own conceptual identity – in approaching more appropriately the psychosocial worlds created by men in their societies. Concepts such as 'appreciation' suggested by Sir Geoffrey Vickers (1965, 1968) no longer require apology. All these steps are apprehended as being within science, which seems more self-consistent if less unified. Science as a method, as an inquiring system, has liberated itself from the domination of the physical sciences, indeed from 'scientism' (Kaplan, 1964; Churchman, 1967).

The appearance of an integrative strategy has shown that science has become able to cope with the reality of wholeness as well as that of elements. So long as it seemed to insist that only elements were real it did violence to a 'truth' intuitively grasped in human experience, as the Gestalt psychologists showed many years ago in the field of perception. More generally and recently, the integrative strategy has emerged in terms of the 'systems' concept (Ashby, 1959).

Russell Ackoff sums it up as follows:

> In the last two decades we have witnessed the emergence of the 'system' as a key concept in scientific research. Systems, of course, have been studied for centuries, but something new has been added. Until recently scientists and engineers tended to treat systems as complexes whose output could be expressed as a simple function of the outputs of the component parts. As a consequence, systems were designed from the inside out. Increasingly researchers have come to deal with systems whose output cannot be expressed as a simple function of component outputs and it has become more productive to treat them holistically and to design them from the outside in (Ackoff, 1959).

The systems concept has had a double origin, for it arose in 'systems engineering' as well as in theoretical biology. The sharing of a common concept has enabled pure and applied science to merge their activities in a way not previously possible. There have been two related effects:

(a) disciplines of a new kind have arisen, for example operational research (sometimes called 'systems analysis'), which are becoming linked to the social sciences (Lawrence, 1964);
(b) these disciplines deal directly with technological and social systems in the complexity in which they exist.

This is a capability that science did not have at an earlier period. It has greatly increased its usefulness to those concerned with the management of human affairs just as the other advances mentioned have reduced the likelihood of its leading them into error.

New Concepts of Policy

If science has been changing so has policy. While the former has become more policy-aware the latter has become more science-aware. They have become 'directively correlated'[1] in response to the increased uncertainties and interdependencies of the contemporary environment. These have had two effects on policy-making which have made it seek to become more 'science-based':

(a) the greater uncertainty requires more future-orientation;
(b) the greater interdependence requires more comprehensiveness.

When the change-rate was slower, policy could be largely corrective, acting after the event. With a faster change-rate, it has had to become more anticipatory, acting before the event. This relates it to planning. The task of government now extends from regulating the present to creating conditions for the future. This entails deciding how resources are to be committed in the future, yet without somehow foreclosing too much, so that this future may take place in one of the more desirable of its alternative forms. Such a task cannot be carried out without an extensive information base which can only be brought into being and maintained through the use of a wide range of sciences. Moreover, this task continuously challenges these sciences to develop new concepts and methods.

In the economic and social fields, the first requirement is a more informed picture of the present, the state of which becomes more unknown the faster and more uneven the change-rate. Disaggregated as well as aggregated statistics and indicators are needed for short-run projections, the identification of high-risk areas, and the separation of the least from the most changing parts of the society. Beyond this, techniques have to be developed for detecting and interpreting emergent social processes and for constructing models of alternative futures.

When the subsystems of society were less interdependent, policies could be more discrete and separate agencies could administer their own programmes with minimum reference to each other. The greater degree of interdependence has changed this situation. Diffuse problems now arise which affect several sections or indeed the whole of society and these problems tend themselves to be interconnected. Examples would be poverty, obsolescence, urban decay, pollution, overpopulation, regional disparity, water and other natural resource management, and intergenerational conflict. The complex perceptions and beliefs that arise about such interconnected areas (rapidly diffused by the media) Michel Chevalier (1967) has called 'meta-problems'. They are less accurately related to the source problems than when these were more bounded and linked to the direct experience of particular groups. Diagnosis is correspondingly more difficult.

Problem-oriented Research Domains

The changed relationship of science and policy and the changes that have been taking place in each have led to the emergence of a new type of scientific activity. This tends to be confused with more familiar types. The spectrum of scientific activities has been thought of as including fundamental or basic research, applied research and development work. The economists have recently added another term: innovation. This refers to the additional activities that must be undertaken before the benefits of R & D can be realized in goods and services effective in the market place. The concept of innovation is also applicable to the non-market sector. If the ends of the spectrum are now clearer something has become blurred in the middle. For some time the term 'problem-oriented research' has been struggling into existence not knowing whether it should be subsumed under applied research or represent something different. The thesis is advanced that it comprises a distinct category whose recognition has central importance for science policy and its social aspects.

If fundamental research is discipline-based, problem-oriented research may be said to be domain-based (McWhinney, 1968). Domain-based inquiry links a group of sciences to a major sector of social concern. The problems are generic rather than specific. They give rise to meta-problems. They require ongoing endeavour leading to cumulations of findings rather than 'solutions'. These findings contribute simultaneously to the advancement of knowledge and to human betterment. The development of a domain is jointly determined by the social and scientific interests concerned. From the policy standpoint such a domain has the characteristics of future-orientation and comprehensiveness. On the scientific side it involves the integrative strategy. Disciplines across the entire range of the physical, biological, and social sciences tend to be drawn in. Their weighting and salience vary enormously between domains, which have very different centres and may evolve very different configurations.

Scientists, professionals, administrators, and political representatives all become involved. The texture of their relationships differs from what it is in fundamental research, where scientific interest predominates, or applied research, where user-interest predominates. The relations of the different actors in a problem-oriented domain is that of collaboration. Bound together by common commitment to the overriding purpose, they have to recognize the complementarity of their contributions and respect each other's authority.

Domain-based problem-oriented research has experienced difficulties not only in securing recognition as a distinct activity but in finding appropriate organizational settings.[2] Novel problems of decision-making and mutual responsibility are posed. These are not well understood and institutions that will allow the necessary experience to be gained still to a large extent await development. This is scarcely surprising since domain-based research represents the confluence or emergent trends in both science and policy.

No systematic attempt has yet been made to describe problem-oriented research in terms of the domain concept or to relate such domains to the discipline-based fields of fundamental research or the user-prescribed missions of applied research. Obviously, one type of work can give rise to the others. If the overall scientific enterprise were to be mapped in domain terms, some fundamental, as well as applied, work would be included in this direction. It is based on a sector-type concept as the most familiar way of thinking in terms of domains (see *Table 1*). Such a listing may serve to disclose the multiplicity and pervasiveness of problem-oriented research domains in the scientific enterprise of a modern society.

The most clearly identifiable and most commonly recognized domains are in the first group centred on a concern with the resources of the biological and physical environment – their discovery and scientific explanation, their cultivation, utilization, and conservation. Medicine and agriculture are the time-honoured members. Natural resources have only belatedly come to be regarded as a comprehensive domain, in contrast to the newcomer – space. In most developed and some developing countries there have been created bodies, governmental, private, or mixed, that overview these domains. A history of the British Research Councils and their changing terms of reference would make an invaluable study in this context, especially if compared with analogous bodies elsewhere – not only in the West but in Eastern Europe, where the Departments as distinct from the Institutes of the Academies of Sciences perform not dissimilar functions.

The next group centres on technology in relation to industry. But in this vast territory concerned with the productive capability of the economy (which gave rise to the classical meaning of applied research) there would appear to be no commonly recognized set of domains. In some European countries technology is perceived as belonging with basic science rather than industry and grouped with it in a Ministry of Science, whereas in Britain the Ministry of Technology and Board of Trade have recently been grouped together, still further emphasizing the separation of applied from basic science which is associated with education in a Ministry of Education and Science. Each of these appreciations has its own validity

TABLE 1 *Problem-oriented research domains*

Domain	*Key programme areas and aspects*
Medicine	Biological sciences related to medicine; biomedical engineering; clinical and epidemiological studies, including psychological and social aspects; design and appraisals of health-care systems and services.
Agriculture	Agricultural sciences and technology; the diffusion of improved practices; the rural economy; psychosocial studies of the changing rural society.
Natural resources	Conservation; recreation; economic aspects; earth sciences; oceanography; social and political regulation; pollution control.
Space	Relevant sciences and technology; uses of space for society; analysis of emergent political issues.
Technology and industry	Several subdomains would be required, type of technology giving one possible basis – constructional, mechanical and automotive, electrical, chemical, electronic, nuclear; but technological considered in relation to economic, market, organizational, and human aspects; these are sociotechnical systems.
Human resources	The development and deployment of the individual educationally, vocationally, etc.; the educational and employment and career systems and their linkage at all phases of the life-cycle; relation to leisure.
Family and household	Relating the biological, psychological, and sociological aspects with those of the economic and material environment.
Community and regional	Similar aspects on the community level of analysis, whether urban or rural, local or regional; the concept of the 'built environment' – the relation of physical to social planning.
Law and society	Linking legal, sociological, and psychological studies of social regulation in all fields; legislation, courts, police, offenders, prisons, and rehabilitation, etc.; civil, industrial, matrimonial law, etc.
Developing countries	Cultural, linguistic, racial, economic problems, etc.; population, food, technological transfer; the multidimensional nature of the development process; relations with advanced countries.
Advanced countries	Including the whole range of 'international studies': political; legal; economic; cultural; technological; organizational, etc. Cross-country comparisons; the multinational corporation, transnational bodies of all types.

but the choice made is likely to have far-reaching effects – of a kind not easy to ascertain. Research that is concerned with discovering new or improving existing products or processes may be classified as applied. Such work is related to the world of specific commodities, of market costs and opportunities. These, however, are making unmanageable the world of social costs, many of the effects of economic growth being dysfunctional for the quality of life. It is recognition of this that seems likely to increase the degree to which technological research becomes fashioned in terms of domains. Such domains would bring together the human and organizational, as well as the economic and technical, aspects of productive enterprise and consider its interdependence with other sectors of society. They would thus provide a context for examining the consequences of positive feedback in what Vickers (1970) has described as a self-exciting system.

The third group, centred on the social sciences, is directly concerned with the quality of life within a society. This has become a prevailing topic in the contemporary world because the second industrial revolution, based on the computer and automation, has simultaneously provided opportunities for its enhancement and threats of its reduction that have not existed before. Domain appreciation is likely to be guided by the recognition of two principles: (a) that the quality of life is affected by the quality of social reality at all system levels (not merely the individual) and in all dimensions of value (not merely the economic); and (b) that welfare and development have become interdependent in the transition to post-industrialism – welfare in its widest connotation of well-being and functional intactness (stability) and development in its widest connotation of growth (change) that is progressive and order-producing rather than regressive and disorder-producing (Trist, 1967).

The last group brings together the three previous groups when societies as wholes, or in any of their major aspects, are compared with each other. This they have increasingly to be, in a world that has reached a new level of interrelatedness and interdependence. Because such comparisons emphasize the culture of particular societies in their historical context this group brings together the social sciences and the humanities. It also involves the identification and appraisal of transnational processes and institutions – a new dimension in 'the order of social magnitude'. This can only be done 'geo-centrically' if multinational teams are involved in the scientific enterprise as much as in the multinational corporation, as Perlmutter (1965) has emphasized.

A first annotation suggests that the relationship between science and society expressed in a problem-oriented research domain is a sensitive indicator of prevailing concerns and values. A scrutiny in terms of resource allocation would confirm this. But the list is incomplete. The area that has consumed more scientific resources than any other among the nations on the winning side in the Second World War has been left out: defence. This is the area that gave rise to the concept of mission. One may ask how far defence research is domain- rather than mission-oriented. Less, perhaps, than one might be inclined to assume, concerned as it is with weapon systems rather than probable forms of war (Erickson, 1970). One may ask also how far defence has dominated the whole field in concept generation as well as in resource consumption, delaying recognition of the distinction between domain and mission.

Despite the ambiguities revealed, there is accumulating evidence that field-determined, generic, problem-oriented research expresses the critical relation between science and society in the transition to post-industrialism. It appears to be so in Eastern European countries as well as in the West; the Academies of Sciences, for example, have formed 'problem-councils' in conjunction with Planning Commissions and State Committees on Science and Technology. This is so also in developing countries making the transition from pre-industrialism to industrialism under the same turbulent conditions in which the advanced countries are concerned with the transition to post-industrialism. A recent UNESCO survey has documented this theme as a world trend (Trist, 1970).

What seems to be required for mapping purposes is a matrix that would relate individuals and supra-individual entities to the main dimensions or sections of a society. An 'entities' list might read as follows: individuals, families, formal organizations, communities, regions, countries, supranational institutions. A dimensions list would comprise the social systems belonging to such sectors as: education, government, health, industry, law, welfare, etc. Such a scheme would permit the examination of how far research on health questions was at the individual or the community level, or how far questions of industry and employment were being looked at throughout the country or regionally.

More than one matrix would be required. A useful one could be constructed in terms of prevailing meta-problems. This would cut across the categories of sectorial analysis. It would be nearer to intuitive perceptions of emergent social processes and values (cf. Emery, 1967).

Social and Technical Development and Innovation

The counterpart at the more concrete level of the fusion of social and scientific interests in a problem-oriented research domain is the action-research programme or project carried out by a research group in collaboration with a client system. The client system may be an industrial firm, a public agency in any field, or a wider authority embracing a large number of these. The research group may contain any mix of disciplines – whatever is appropriate to the task in hand.

The strategic significance of this type of work derives from the extent to which new institutions have to be built and old ones renewed during a time of social transition as great as the present. Governments now intervene in the operations of society to an extent previously unknown. New schemes need piloting; their operations need monitoring and evaluating. There is a growing demand in the field of social action for the equivalent of industrial development work and also of product innovation in the sense of the diffusion of a proven pilot throughout the wider system for which it is intended.

Much of this work is technological as well as social, i.e. sociotechnical in the sense of the concept originally introduced in the Tavistock studies of the British mining industry (Trist *et al.*, 1963). It may involve not only the collaborative design of pilot schemes but 'institution-building' in the widest sense to engage the key interest groups in a society. A project that exemplifies an extension of this type of work to the overall societal level has for some years been taking place in Norway, becoming known as the Norwegian Industrial Democracy Project (Emery & Thorsrud, 1969). Sociotechnical experiments originally sponsored by a joint committee of the Federation of Employers and the Federation of Trade Unions have led to the formation of a National Participation Council and a Parliamentary Commission on Industrial Democracy concerned with the diffusion of new principles of job design throughout Norwegian industry.

The increasingly unregulable world that science has been bringing into existence can best be brought back into a more regulated state by applying the methods of science to the change processes occurring within it. This entails engaging in social or operational experiments of many different kinds, but always sanctioned by those concerned. In this way errors and unintended effects are more likely to be picked up before it is too late. So far as all participate, all will learn and the values of science will be diffused into the society, which will itself embody the social aspects of its science policies. But this can only come about in so far as key actors from all four estates collaborate in fashioning the appreciations of what may best be undertaken in the critical research domains.

BASIC MODES OF RESEARCH ORGANIZATION AND THEIR COMPLEMENTARITY

The Basic Types and Their Varieties

The increasing extent to which policy and social research are becoming interrelated, in the ways which have been described, is affecting the character and role of research organizations. Three main types may be distinguished in terms of 'output mix'. Each has a distinctive pattern. They will be referred to as Types A (profession-based), B (discipline-based), and C (domain-based) respectively:[3]

Type A (profession-based)

Centres of professional social science activity, with associated research and development facilities to undertake work on immediate practical problems. These secure the use of expert knowledge by winning expert power – through demonstrating the relevance of their findings to the missions of their sponsors.

These centres are located within user-organizations (such as the Home Office Research Unit in Britain), or constitute consulting groups under contract to them (such as the Société d'économie et de mathématiques appliquées in France). Lacking them, user-organizations remain without agents able to identify areas of social science knowledge relevant to their problems. They are also without social science professionals in continuous contact with administrators. Research problems are determined by client needs, though real and apparent needs are often difficult to distinguish. What is most deeply required is far from always what is most urgently requested. Working through a re-interpretation of the presenting problem while the constraints of the situation are more accurately assessed involves a process of mutual learning between client and research worker.

Such work expresses what may be termed a *research/service* 'mix'.

Type B (discipline-based)

Centres of basic research associated with major teaching facilities. Centres of Type B are the opposite of, and complementary to, those of Type A. They advance the frontiers of fundamental knowledge while ensuring its reproduction in the next generation.

They are located within universities, as autonomous departments based on particular disciplines (such as psychology and sociology) and undertake both undergraduate and graduate training. Here, research problems are more determined by the needs of theory and method or may represent attempts to explore and establish new fields of inquiry. In this way the cognitive structuring of the world becomes changed for men in their societies.

Such work expresses a *research/teaching* 'mix'.

Type C (domain-based)

Centres of applied research associated with advanced research training.

Centres of Type C may be regarded as a resultant of Types A and B. They supply the necessary link between them, being the intermediate bodies between user-organizations and orthodox university departments. They change the appreciation of what has become critical in the relations of men and their environments.

They may be located within the boundaries of universities and related to several Type B departments (such as the Institute for Social Research of the University of Michigan), or outside them as independent institutes (such as the Institute of Preventive Medicine in Leiden). They may be supported by public or private sources or a mixture of both. They are problem-centred and interdisciplinary, but focus on generic rather than specific problems. They accept professional as well as scientific responsibility for the projects they undertake. They contribute both to theoretical development and to the improvement of practice.

Such work expresses a *research/application* 'mix'.

The criteria that differentiate the three types are summarized in *Table 2*.

TABLE 2 *Characteristics of main types of research organization*

Types of work		Type of setting	
	In user- or consulting organizations	In university teaching departments	In special institutes in or outside universities
Source of problem	Specific client needs	Needs of theory and method	General 'field' needs
Level of problem	Concrete	Abstract	Generic
Activity mix	Research/service	Research/teaching	Research/application
Disciplinary mix	Multiple	Single	Interrelated
Overall pattern	Type A (profession-based)	Type B (discipline-based)	Type C (domain-based)

The types form an interdependent system; no one can be fully effective alone, the feedback of each into the others being critical for both the development and the utilization of the social sciences.

The boundaries of A and B can extend into C, and those of C into either A or B, or both. If a distinction is necessary conceptually, overlap is desirable in practice in activities and staff. Many existing research organizations show idiomatic combinations of the basic types: A & B; A & C; B & C; A, B, & C. Examples that include all are professional schools associated with universities, more particularly as these have developed in the United States. Such schools are inherently inter- and multidisciplinary, combining teaching with basic, domain-based, and more specifically applied forms of research and with demonstration practice. Yet schools of administration and business, medicine, engineering, architecture and planning, education, etc., experience much conflict through failing completely to recognize the presence of the different mixes. They do not always place equal value on their distinctive contributions, or organize themselves appropriately for their different requirements. To embody this capability is a key attribute in a multipurpose organization concerned with research, teaching, and the provision of service. Of special interest are the multi-disciplinary schools of applied behavioural science recently recommended by the Joint Survey Committee on the Behavioral and Social Sciences (BASS) in the United States.[4]

Several varieties of research unit occur in each of the main types. These are set out in *Table 3*. Though most of the terms are self-explanatory, one or two need brief comment. By internal agencies, Type A1, are meant

TABLE 3 *Varieties of research unit in relation to main types*

Main type	*Varieties*
the research/service mix user-organizations Type A (profession-based)	1. Internal agencies 2. Directly controlled establishments 3. Consulting organizations
the research/teaching mix university departments Type B (discipline-based)	1. Predoctoral programmes 2. Postdoctoral programmes (basic) 3. Postdoctoral programmes (contract)
the research/application mix special institutes Type C (domain-based)	1. University-based organizations 2. Independent organizations 3. National or transnational organizations (shared costly facility) 4. National or transnational organizations (shared routine facility)

headquarters research and development groups close to centres of policy-making. These are concerned with identifying problems rather than with carrying out investigations. They may initiate exploratory or pilot schemes themselves and undertake urgent, short-run inquiries. Anything more massive, basic, or longer range would be handed over – to one of their own directly controlled research establishments or to an outside consulting organization, Types A2 and A3; to a postdoctoral contract programme in a university, Type B3; or to a Type C organization.

National and transnational institutes, Type C3 (shared costly facility), have been available to the natural sciences for some time, institutes for nuclear physics such as CERN are an example. The computer is bringing them into existence for the social sciences. National data banks are beginning to be established and computer programme collections to be made using the most advanced equipment and software skills. National organizations of Type C4 (shared routine facility) came into existence in the social sciences to collect and analyse statistical data, e.g. the census, social surveys, etc. International facilities of these types are appearing. Type C3 and Type C4 organizations, though national or international in scope, are not necessarily government controlled, even if government financed. They may be funded from several sources, largely private. Their functional independence is a matter requiring the most careful consideration. Their establishment, as a priority, in the main regions of the developing world, was recommended by the UNESCO Round Table on Social Research Policy and Organization recently held in Denmark.[5]

The Research/Service Mix: Type A (Profession-based)

Type A centres possess special capability in initiating inquiries felt to have user relevance. They tend therefore to become influential in securing utilization of results. Individual departments of government are increasingly being accorded social science budgets to develop such centres. They require freedom of decision in respect of the type of work undertaken and the type of technical assistance sought – internal or external. The practice of the more advanced industries in the public, no less than in the private, sector is based on such an attitude towards technological research. Though needing very considerable strengthening as regards social research this attitude is now beginning to spread within all developed countries.

Two very strong reasons may be advanced for linking Type A centres with the operating organizations directly concerned with their activities:

(a) only when made responsible for its own research and development can an operating organization develop the scientific outlook imperative under conditions of increasing technological and environmental change; the future adaptability of the agency or enterprise lies more than ever before in its R & D.

(b) now that so many government departments, no less than industrial enterprises, have developed gigantic operational functions, the scale and heterogeneity of their tasks compose an internal world, large and various enough for a research and development organization to belong to it and still retain 'many degrees of freedom'.

The more such organizations are separated off and assembled under a central research and development authority the greater the tendency to stunt the growth of each, to inhibit integration with administration, and to create an outsize scientific bureaucracy. At least this is so under conditions of the advanced countries. By contrast, in developing countries where scientific resources are scarce to create a single competent and viable establishment close to the centres of power may often represent the optimal strategy of choice. This is especially so when these countries are small.

Yet many people continue to feel that the independence of the scientist is threatened in any directly controlled research establishment. Autonomous research councils as exemplified in the British tradition provide in their belief both the necessary and the sufficient conditions for the development of science in relation to government. It is our belief also that autonomous research councils are necessary. Indeed we advocate two types – the *basic* and the *applied* in the sense of domain-based – but in relation to Type B and Type C problems and centres. With regard to Type A problems and centres the nature of the relationship between user-organization and research establishment is such as to place the advantage with direct linkage. Nevertheless, this advantage has to be sacrificed when interference from the executive branch for reasons either of ideology or expediency precludes any rational modification of policy by scientific findings. The scientist has no option but to resign when policy becomes counter-scientific. This issue is to be distinguished from that concerning classified research in areas where security is essential in government for reasons of the national interest or in private enterprise for reasons of product or market advantage. What is unacceptable now is the constraining of activities and the restriction of publication in the name of security when danger is negligible or even non-existent. Such considerations apart, the wider acceptance of a scientific outlook in an increasing number of societies is undoubtedly strengthening the position of scientists inside organizations. This is not to say that for many purposes outside consulting groups are not also necessary, or indeed to be preferred, or to deny that by the mere fact of their existence they strengthen the hand of the men inside. Their complementary role will be discussed below. What outside groups cannot do is to provide transactional continuity at the science–policy interface. This can only be done from the inside.

The utilization of scientific knowledge within a user-organization concerns the relations between three types of people:

(a) administrators (managers)
(b) professional practitioners (technical staffs)
(c) scientific workers in associated research and development agencies and establishments.

Effectively to relate administrators and researchers requires the presence of a third-party group – professional practitioners. These are the medium through which transformation of knowledge and purpose, necessary for communications, takes place, in both directions. Though this principle has been well established for the physical and biological sciences, through the functions carried out by many types of engineering and medical personnel, social science professionals have been slow to emerge in organizational contexts. This has delayed the pace of advance.

The most fruitful developments cannot take place unless professional practitioners and researchers, as well as administrators, can report to the top policy-making level, where the political world enters. The four estates (scientific, professional, administrative, and political) require to be in mutual engagement at the 'institutional' rather than simply at the 'operational' level of management (cf. Parsons, 1960). But it remains the exception for any social scientist, other than an economist, to gain access at this level. All the main reports, both national and international, made during the decade of the sixties on the use of the social sciences have stressed the need to include members of other disciplines in what Bertram Gross (1966) has called the Central Guidance Cluster.

When a user-organization is new to research, long-range or highly specialized projects, in which generic or basic problems are dominant, are best contracted out to universities or independent centres. A user-organization becomes more likely to develop effective research establishments of its own (Type A2), as distinct from internal agencies (Type A1), if it first collaborates with experienced outside organizations. As learning takes place, the boundary of what it is able to do internally is pushed back.

Type A1, the internal headquarters agency, is most easily thought of as a relatively small group of about six rather senior people, including the head of social research and development in the organization as a whole who would act as chief social science adviser at the top policy-making level. Such a group would be concerned with problem identification and appreciation, the strategy of investigation, and the application and dissemination of findings, rather than with very much in the way of fieldwork – except on a pilot scale. They would spend much of their time with administrators and other professionals. As distinct entities, such agencies would be expected to appear only in very large organizations (whether in government or outside it). Very few units of this kind, explicitly based on the social sciences (apart from economics), yet exist. Nevertheless, they made their debut (not unsuccessfully) during the Second World War in the fighting services and in certain branches of civil government in several countries. One may recall the series of substantial innovations brought about by the Directorate of Psychiatry and the Directorate of Selection of Personnel in the British Army (Rees, 1945). A minimum establishment is suggested in *Table 4*. It is doubtful if this group could profitably be larger than twelve, or fifteen at the very most. The ideal in this context is a face-to-face group, small enough for all members to keep in personal contact but large enough to permit absentees, for some will always be away on assignments, often abroad.

TABLE 4 *Internal agency: Type A1 (minimum size)*

*Scientific staff**	*Role*	*Number*
Senior	Director and chief social science adviser	1
	Deputy director	1
Middle	Research officers each responsible for a problem area	4
Total		6

*Junior staff not included in a headquarters group

Type A2, the directly controlled establishment, is much more of a field investigation group, though in smaller organizations it would tend to include also the headquarters function of Type A1. To be viable, such a group must be large enough to maintain a planned programme and at the same time have the resources to launch new developments, to meet emergencies, and to cope with its own growth and turnover. A director with some two or three project leaders, and a total staff of about fifteen, is the type of set-up minimally envisaged (*Table 5*). Though this number

TABLE 5 *Directly controlled establishment: Type A2 (minimum size)*

Scientific staff	*Role*	*Number*
Senior	Director	1
	Project leaders	3
Middle	Fieldworkers	4
Junior	Fieldworkers	7
Total		15

could easily extend upwards, the effectiveness and stability of a group much smaller in size would be questionable except in an early stage of development. Too large a group would also be questionable, because the range of problems (at this level of concreteness) could easily become too great to preserve cohesion. A second establishment might preferably be created when there are more than six project leaders and numbers overall exceed thirty; the less hierarchy the better.

Centres of Type A2 are increasing noticeably at the present time, though many are new and precariously small. The danger is that too many of them will be confined to trivia by constraining terms of reference, through the absence of a protecting and opportunity-creating A1 unit with the necessary leverage to secure relevant assignments.

Type A3, outside consulting organizations, in order to survive independently require to be larger, more on the scale suggested for the special institutes, with a scientific staff of not less than thirty-five. We are thinking here not so much of organizations concerned with applying established techniques as those concerned with innovation. Such organizations may sometimes, with advantage, lie within the framework of another organization much larger still and concerned with more routine work, but only if this itself is in a state that is giving rise to innovation. Otherwise the stability gained will be offset by the restrictions imposed, as is not uncommon in the field of market research.

Because of their independence, outside consulting organizations can exercise considerable power in assisting client organizations to develop a greater innovative capability and to undergo and implement change, qualities increasingly essential in adapting to a world of rising uncertainty. A number of these organizations, such as the Institute for Applied Behavioral Science (NTL) and the Organization for Social and Technical Innovation in the US, display a *network character*. They often have a large proportion of part-time staff who hold appointments in universities. They have the capability to mobilize dispersed resources to form task forces (temporary systems) for dealing with special problems. This is becoming increasingly necessary. Required resource combinations are far from likely always to be found or permanently maintained in one place. Network organizations have special competence in operating internationally and in forming consortia. All this, of course, is not peculiar to Type A; universities in a number of countries have recently become more enterprising along these lines. Nevertheless, an organizational philosophy of sharing parts across boundaries is still relatively new.

Some Type A work inevitably takes on a more generic quality so that the organizations involved acquire Type C characteristics. Professional ethics and an understanding of the nature of the collaborative relationship in taking joint responsibility with client systems are critical attributes for such organizations. As only large organizations are likely to develop competent in-house facilities, the role of outside groups, as change agents for medium-sized and smaller organizations of all kinds, is a key one.

There are also many circumstances in which the best results are obtained through the collaboration of an internal and external resource group – even in the largest organizations. This pattern is gaining ground when strategic questions are involved and profound organizational changes are required. This approach has become common in applications of the social sciences to large technologically advanced industry in the United States. The Public Administration Division of the United Nations is currently employing it in relation to problems of development administration (UN, 1969). Government departments in a number of countries have begun to use it with increasing freedom in the last few years.

The Research/Teaching Mix: Type B (Discipline-based)

Many research problems of a basic kind (Type B2) are best pursued entirely within a university framework, the continuous development of fundamental research being a necessary complement to Type A activities in user-organizations and consulting groups. Fundamental research is greatly enhanced by the availability of internal funds. If solely dependent on external funds provided by foundations, research councils, or other contracting agencies, dysfunctional constraints enter from factors of competition, the predictions of review boards, and the general lines of science policy, however good this may be from an overall standpoint. It is easy to be 'out of programme' and it is often difficult for originality to be recognized outside the immediate circle of an investigator, especially when his project is in a formative stage. Thinking time, probes, and pilot runs are hard to finance externally, while the costs of preparing elaborate proposals and a good deal of writing up are notoriously difficult to recover. External funds are necessary to meet the expense of projects or programmes of any magnitude. The two types of funding are complementary. Now that external funds have become more plentiful in many countries, the invaluable contribution of internal funds and the need to provide them should not be overlooked.

The highest priority in the short run is, in almost all countries outside the United States, for universities to increase and improve the supply of social science researchers. Those now available fall short of even present requirements, certainly in quantity and too often in quality. Two points may be made:

(a) It is neither possible nor desirable that more than a proportion (however substantial) of those who subsequently enter social science careers should, as undergraduates, have pursued far, or even at all, any of the major disciplines of the social sciences. Many of the potentially best students come to know about the social sciences only quite late. The priority development in the universities as regards the social sciences needs to be in graduate studies. The United States is the only country where organized graduate education has become an established tradition in the social sciences, though in some European countries a first degree that takes five or six years gives a solid foundation. Needed are intensive make-up courses of one year for those with some undergraduate preparation, and of two years for those with none. These would enable a basic theoretical and methodological competence to be acquired rapidly by mature students with a commitment to research and proven academic ability. The Social Science Research Council has been encouraging such developments in Britain.

(b) Such courses should include opportunities to acquire practical experience as well as book knowledge. This may be done by providing 'internships' or attachments for periods of, say, three months during the summer vacation – in Type A centres prepared to offer facilities for practical training. This approach needs extensive development and provides scope for a great deal of innovation.

Because the advancement of knowledge and the extension of practice in the social sciences are interdependent, universities need to provide professional as well as research training. As such developments occur, they will change the size and the character of a number of social science departments and greatly increase the amount of social science taught in schools of education, social work, medicine, law, business and public administration, engineering, and technology. To his surprise the writer found in a recent study of American universities that the number of faculties in professional schools with social science backgrounds already exceeded those in professional schools with natural science backgrounds. This trend foreshadows the emergence of the post-industrial society.

Once formal graduate courses are established the next step is to ensure that extensive predoctoral research programmes of Type B1 are organized so that those proceeding to research careers undergo a thorough research apprenticeship leading to the establishment of a definite professional and scientific identity. When this has been established students become more easily capable of entering into relations with those in other disciplines and of developing in themselves the broader outlook and competence that are a condition of effective participation in interdisciplinary programmes (Sanford, 1963).

A sketch is made in *Table 6* of the type of establishment likely to be minimally required by a university department concerned with a single social science discipline. On the teaching side there would be graduate courses of two kinds – basic and professional, an undergraduate honours school, and other undergraduate courses given as part requirements in other departments. On the research side there would be a number of PhD

TABLE 6 *University department: Type B (minimum size)*

<table>
<tr><th>Scientific staff</th><th>Role</th><th>Teaching emphasis</th><th>Research emphasis</th><th>Total</th></tr>
<tr><td>Senior</td><td>Departmental chairman</td><td colspan="2">1</td><td></td></tr>
<tr><td></td><td>Other professors, readers, or programme directors (full professors in US terms)</td><td>2</td><td>1</td><td>4</td></tr>
<tr><td>Middle</td><td>Lecturers and postdoctoral researchers (associate professors in US terms)</td><td>3</td><td>3</td><td>6</td></tr>
<tr><td>Junior</td><td>Assistant lecturers and predoctoral researchers (assistant professors in US terms)</td><td>–</td><td>20</td><td>20</td></tr>
<tr><td>Total</td><td></td><td>5·5</td><td>24·5</td><td>30</td></tr>
</table>

candidates to supervise, various postdoctoral projects in basic research and others of a contract character.

This total set of activities could scarcely be carried out by fewer than thirty people, some of whom would be more concerned with research and others with the teaching side, but flexible and interchangeable according to interest and career phase. Included are a number of advanced graduate students assisting in the teaching as well as completing PhD degrees. Multiple chairs are essential. The basic social science disciplines such as sociology, economics, and psychology encompass territories of knowledge too vast to be mastered in depth by one man ('the professor'). The number of senior staff should be large enough to enable several of the main branches of such a discipline to be taught and researched at the highest level. The boundary areas should also be developed so that each department can relate itself to its neighbours.

An adequate level of non-academic support staff of all kinds as well as of technical facilities and libraries is of paramount importance. The shortfall of such provisions in most universities is woeful.

Given proper administrative and technical backup, a staff of 30 of the type described, with a heavy complement of juniors, could maintain a considerable research enterprise while at the same time meeting the needs of a sizable student body. Let us assume that those deployed during a given year with teaching emphasis give two-thirds of their time to teaching and one-third to research, and that those deployed with research emphasis reverse these proportions. The teaching resources available overall should be able to manage 150 full-time students – an undergraduate honours school of 75 and a graduate school also of 75, some 50 of whom would be taking conversion courses. If the undergraduate curriculum covered three years and the graduate curriculum two, each class group would be small enough to permit seminar as well as lecture methods. In addition, we will postulate 100 part-time students, whether undergraduate or graduate, committed in various degrees to courses in other fields and count them as the equivalent of another 50 full-time students. Overall, the teaching effort of the staff of 30 would be distributed among 200 students (full-time equivalents). This is a more generous faculty-student ratio than a norm of one to ten would prescribe. The difference represents an investment in the development of junior staff at the immediately pre- or immediately postdoctoral level, none of whom need teach for more than one-third of their time. This would permit a rapid development of an experienced research force trained to the highest standard in close contact with more senior people. As their careers developed they would enable the social science enterprise to expand both inside and outside the university.

Yet many people outside the US, where much larger faculties and student bodies are common, would think of such a department as relatively large rather than as relatively small – at least in the social sciences. *Table 7*

TABLE 7 *The social sciences in an American university as illustrated by the University of California, Los Angeles (1966)*

	Full professors	*Other faculty*	*Total faculty*
Basic social science departments			
Anthropology	12	22	34
Economics	12	25	37
Linguistics	10	20	30
Political science	11	29	40
Psychology	20	75	95
Sociology	10	30	40
Total	75	201	276
Professional schools			
Business administration	30	59	89
Education	33	41	74
Psychiatry	6	76	82
Public health	24	98	122
Social welfare	4	24	28
Total	97	298	395

gives the faculty strength in the social science departments, pure and applied, in an American university (the figures do not include a number of temporary staff or PhD candidates working as teaching assistants). The multidisciplinary professional schools deriving from or extensively dependent on the social sciences have faculties roughly twice the size of the basic departments. Among these psychology is the exception – but it is a double department, bio-physical on one hand, bio-social on the other. Among the professional schools social welfare has remained relatively undeveloped. His experience in the particular university convinced the writer that large faculties, much larger than that proposed in the minimum model, can function cohesively. The danger is in the sub-threshold department that knows that it cannot responsibly develop the main features of its field of knowledge. A university social science department needs 'critical mass' and 'requisite variety'.

The Research/Application Mix: Type C (Domain-based)

The 'special institutes' constitute a distinct genus. They are more problem-centred than orthodox university departments, and in this sense more applied. But the problems they are concerned with are more general than those taken up by research and development groups inside organizations or by consultants. The results they obtain are intended to be fed back into basic research. Being problem-centred, their work tends in varying degrees to become interdisciplinary. It provides test conditions for scientific innovation. In view of the particular significance in the present state of the social sciences of research on field-determined generic problems, the fostering of special institutes is crucial for future developments.

Some organizations of this kind serve a useful but transitional purpose. The value of this group is that they are expendable. Many exploratory missions are best carried out by temporary systems. No questions of tenure or career investment need arise; for those concerned the experience is an episode in which unusually high risks can be taken.

Other such organizations develop more enduring capabilities. A characteristic of the latter group is that they tend to be the result of complex trends which converged in a particular setting at a particular time. This gives each such organization an idiomatic quality which is hard to reproduce and tends to endure if the need that brought it into existence endures. Relative freedom of institutional position increases adaptiveness to the changing demands of emergent problems.

Given the rate and complexity of scientific development, new organizations of this type will always be needed, whatever their durability. In the older sciences distinctive competence is often associated with an area of intense specialization. In the newer it is more apt to be associated with a special range of problem areas. The variety of functions, however, is considerable, as is size. Some examples are given in *Table 8* which show that institutes of many kinds with Type C properties exist in all countries where the social sciences are at all developed. They are being asked for in countries where they are not (such as Ecuador). Yet nowhere are they

TABLE 8 *Examples of special institutes*

Type C1: university-based	*Type C2: independent*
The Social Research Organization of the National University, Australia	The European Co-ordination Centre for Social Science Research & Documentation, UNESCO, Austria
The Centre for Culture and Technology (University of Toronto), Canada	The Danish National Institute for Social Research, Denmark
Centres for various branches of Social Research, École pratique des hautes études, France	The Institute for Preventive Medicine, Holland
The Gokhale Institute of Politics and Economics, India	The Demographic Training Centre (UN supported), India.
The Institute of Social Research (National University), Mexico	The Institute for Economic Growth, India
The Institute of Psychological and Social Studies (University of Dakar), Senegal	The Institute for Social Research, Norway
The Institute of Criminology (Cambridge University), UK	The Institute for Philosophy and Sociology (Academy of Sciences), Poland
The Centre for the Analysis of Conflict (London University), UK	The National Institute for Economic and Social Research, UK
The Institute for Social Research (University of Michigan), US	The Tavistock Institute of Human Relations, UK
The Management Science Center (University of Pennsylvania), US	The Brookings Institution, US
The Center for Urban Studies (Wayne State University), US	The Institute for the Future, US
The Social Research Centre (University of Munster), West Germany	The National Institute for Mental Health, US
	Instituto Caribe de Anthropologia y Sociologia (Fundacion La Salle), Venezuela

fully developed, even in American universities, so strong are departmental traditions.

Some of the social science sections of the Academies of Sciences in Eastern Europe would appear to constitute one of the most advanced versions. They express a C-B combination, which may be an innovation of wide import. This combination also characterizes the Social Research Organization of the Australian National University and many of the groups belonging to the École pratique des hautes études. These institutions reflect the need, paramount under certain conditions, to nourish a key research capability associated with advanced training and protect it from the dysfunctional distractions to which ordinary university settings give rise when they become mass undertakings. Rand-type centres in the US constitute another innovation, with a C-A combination, as does the recently established Institute for the Future. Organizations such as the Institut national de la statistique et des études économiques (INSÉÉ) and the Institut national d'études démographiques (INÉD) in France are centred on C but include B as well as A. They have been learning as they go along how to manage this immense range. Some institutes in India and some of those in Latin America are similar in form, however short of qualified and experienced personnel.

Another class of special institutes provides analyses of and commentary on economic and social trends and processes independently of those made by government bodies. Examples are the National Institute for Economic and Social Research in Britain, the Brookings Institution in the US, and the Institute for Economic Growth in India. *Table 8* also contains examples of multipurpose institutes such as the Danish National Institute for Social Research and the Institute for Social Research in Norway, or the centres mentioned in Senegal and Venezuela. These are not uncommon in smaller countries and may be initiated by government, private interests, or a combination of both.

Some very large organizations that include the social sciences have appeared in the medical field at national level – the Institute for Preventive Medicine in Holland and the National Institute for Mental Health in the US. A number of attempts have also been made with UN support to establish regional 'growth centres' in the social sciences in the developing countries in South East Asia, Latin America, and Africa. Several of the organizations in *Table 8* exemplify the class of special institutes that concentrates on a broad problem area – conflict, crime, urban affairs, technology and culture, etc. The Institute for Social Research and the Tavistock have evolved into a cluster of related centres – an indication of the flexibility of the underlying pattern. The consortium function is illustrated by the Social Research Centre at Munster which co-ordinates groups associated with several German universities. To develop this function at the international level is the aim of the UNESCO Vienna Centre.

An independent Type C institute in Britain, such as the Tavistock Institute of Human Relations, finds itself pulled too far in the A direction. This is not simply for financial reasons. It is frequently difficult to know beforehand how far certain Type A projects may develop Type C properties that are more critical for the advance of social science than do certain conventional projects which start out as Type C activities. Open-endedness and open-mindedness are both required in this regard.

University institutes are apt to be pulled too far in the B direction. An incompatibility exists between the research/teaching and the research/application mix unless teaching can be integrated into ongoing programmes. Commitment to long-range high-risk scientific missions which involve groups do not harmonize with complying with the regulations that surround degrees (which require proof of the competence of individuals) unless special provisions are instituted which are supported by the wider university system.

To add to a basic academic competence effective training, not only in research operations but in taking responsibility in the field, a large number of research workers in their immediately postdoctoral years and also a proportion of those in predoctoral programmes need to pursue their studies in centres of this type (especially C1 and C2). A minimum number of such centres is necessary for developing a country's social science capability, especially as regards the type of social science that is policy related.

Customarily, Type C institutes undertake a mixture of contract and grant-aided work supported by a variety of public and private sources. To be effective, they require financial stability. They need a measure of basic support over and above that provided by ordinary research grants or contract fees. Too few of them have this. Because of their innovative character and their responsibility for advanced training, they incur high costs. They pose awkward problems to grant-giving bodies. Private universities can sometimes nourish them from internal funds. Research councils and foundations are apt, at times mistakenly, to stop short of providing institutional support. Recognition of the need to provide such support is growing. Recent changes in the direction of providing institution support have taken place in federal science policy in the US (Trist, 1970).

To use their 'requisite variety', Type C institutes need to be of considerable, though not necessarily vast, size. A research staff of thirty-five would appear to constitute a balanced number for a small institute (*Table 9*).

TABLE 9 *A smaller type special institute: C*

Number in project team	*Number of projects*	*Scientific staff*			*Total staff*
		senior	*middle*	*junior*	
1	5	3	2	–	5
2	4	4	–	4	8
3	3	3	3	3	9
4	2	2	1	5	8
5	1	1	1	3	5
Total	15	13	7	15	35

Another critical point is reached with a staff level of sixty to seventy. This enables a number of project teams of varying sizes and complexions to pursue simultaneously a range of problems, each of which has a bearing on the others. Under such conditions sufficient resources are available to concentrate forces on critical issues, to re-deploy as new avenues open up without undoing ongoing work, and to carry, without undue strain, the high level of waste and uncertainty associated with complex research undertakings. Where much higher levels of staff are contemplated (*Table 10*), an alternative that merits consideration is that of creating more than one establishment rather than a single organization, since the latter might be so big that its innovative capability would be endangered by bureaucratization – other than in special circumstances.

TABLE 10 *A larger type special institute: C*

Number in project team	*Number of projects*	*Scientific staff*			*Total staff*
		senior	*middle*	*junior*	
1	5	5	2	–	7
2	4	4	–	4	8
3	3	3	3	3	9
4	5	5	3	12	20
5	4	4	4	12	20
6	3	4	3	9	16
7	2	4	4	6	14
Total	26	29	19	46	94

Circumstances justifying much larger size include the requirements of Type C3 and C4 organizations concerned with gathering and analysing social and economic data on a national or international scale, and establishing computer-linked networks of data archives and retrieval systems. For example, in 1966 INSÉÉ in France had 3769 employees in 18 centres of whom 246 were scientific professionals. The Indian Institute of Statistics employed some 2000 workers part or full time, of whom 500 were interviewers.

General Characteristics

The overall pattern of basic institutional forms that has been described is a general model. These basic forms, their varieties, and their combinations, which can become exceedingly idiomatic, appear in the context of widely differing educational systems and in relation to scientific 'infrastructures' of widely differing efficacy. Nevertheless, development of the social sciences requires certain underlying structural conditions and the recognition of certain key relations. It is these that the model attempts to represent.

Decision-making structures are likely to be, and should be, different for the research/application, research/teaching, and research/service mixes.

(a) In the research/application mix the most effective choices are likely to be the outcome of complex 'appreciations' which grow up between groups of social scientists, client organizations, and representatives of broader sections of the society. Such processes could lead to the establishment of a number of applied research councils (titles will vary) concerned with developing strategic relations between the social sciences and major sections of a society. The emergence of 'problem councils' in conjunction with the Academies of Sciences in several Eastern European countries may be noted in this context, while in Western Europe, commissions, boards, or committees covering several broad social domains have been established by bodies concerned with the overall planning and utilization of the social sciences.

(b) The research/teaching mix would appear to benefit from the existence of bodies responsible for continuously reviewing the most promising avenues of fundamental research, provided they guide rather than instruct those responsible for initiating projects. Critical judgements here involve what Sir Peter Medawar (1967) has called the 'art of the soluble'. But there is less consensus about what the next set of feasible problems might be in the social as compared with the natural sciences, and a corresponding need to encourage alternative approaches.

(c) Paradoxically, unfashionable innovations may be most effectively nurtured by user-interests concerned with the research/service mix. Some of the most promising new ideas arise in this area. They do not consume much in the way of special resources in their early stages. They may go on quietly as an adjunct of service until enough headway has been made for support to be sought in terms of one of the other two mixes. This is the common way in clinical research.

Developments have been held back by the confusion that has persisted concerning the relations of pure and applied research. These are different in the social and the natural sciences. In the latter the required data can be abstracted from their natural settings to a far greater extent than in the social sciences. For except in special areas, the social scientist must gain access to his material in its natural setting in ways acceptable to those concerned. This means that engagement in problem-oriented research represents a major strategy for advancing the knowledge base in the social sciences.

The effective development of the social sciences towards the needs of the future requires the establishment of genuinely programmatic research, sustained over long periods on carefully selected themes, by institutes with the stability, scale, and 'requisite variety' of resources to enable them to commit their members to such objectives. For reasons concerning both the state of the social sciences and the needs of society a good proportion of these programmes should be in areas of generic field-determined problem-oriented research. At present there is too great a dispersion of research effort in small and unstable organizations. This has resulted in a random accumulation of projects rather than an evolving cumulation of findings. One cause has been the persistence of a tradition of academic individualism among research workers. Echoing this, grant-giving bodies have tended to prefer the apparently reduced risk of backing a large number of small projects to the apparently increased risk of giving support to a limited number of large but strategically selected programmes. A main task of social science policy would be to create the 'enabling conditions' for strategic programmes to be undertaken.

CHANGING THE SCIENTIFIC VALUE SYSTEM

Dysfunctional Persistence of Academic Individualism

The total set of conditions postulated as 'requisite' for the most favourable overall development of the social sciences is not yet in being anywhere in the world. Considering the scale and rate of rising demand, one may ask why things are not further advanced. One factor is that a serious mismatch exists between certain features of the Western academic tradition and the needs of contemporary societies to develop a higher level of social science capability. Yet it was this very tradition that allowed universities in the wake of the Renaissance to establish the right, without interference from church or state, to conduct free inquiry in all fields of scholarship. Without the establishment of this right, first the physical and then the biological sciences could never have developed. Indeed, the foundations of the social sciences themselves would never have been laid.

Three features require examination: (a) the privilege of free inquiry was granted to scholars and embodied in the autonomy of their universities at a price – their dissociation from the larger society; (b) within the autonomous but segregated university the privilege of free inquiry was vested in the right of the individual scholar to pursue his subject in his own way; (c) the right to pursue one's subject in one's own way was not to be granted lightly, indeed only to those who could prove themselves in the eyes of established scholars; hence the *rite de passage* of the doctorate, the individual character of the thesis being sacrosanct, even though the theme required professorial approval.

So long as the advancement of knowledge depended on the separation of pure science from its possible applications and on the personal contributions of a relatively small number of outstanding scholars, the tradition of academic individualism represented an adaptive value on which to found the organization of science. This phase has now been *dépassé,* to use Sartre's term. New values, which have yet to be identified, must be sought.

The situation is more extensively recognized in the natural than in the social sciences. In the former the interpenetration of science and technology has long been taken for granted, as has the need for group as well as individual effort, and for large-scale as well as small-scale research, continued over long periods. It is in the social sciences that the tradition of academic individualism dies hardest.

The Nature of the Required Changes

What is the nature of the changes required? They would seem to involve a fundamental shift:

(a) The right of the individual scholar to pursue freely what he elects to pursue will remain, wherever access to the social field is not a critical issue. It can remain also so long as the complexity and scale of the problem are such that they can be encompassed by a single mind. An increasing number of the key problems, however, in many of the areas with which the social sciences are becoming concerned raise critical issues of access and of pluralistic contribution.

(b) This means that the tradition of academic individualism can no longer play the role of 'the leading part'[6] in a philosophy of the social sciences. It cannot for this reason provide the basic criterion on which the organizations necessary for the development of the social sciences can be built. It can play the role only of a subordinate part.

To accept this is a difficult shift in perspective and values for the present body of social scientists.

Several corollaries follow:

(a) If engagement in applied research of the generic kind represents a fundamental strategy for advancing the knowledge base, then the social science 'university' must find a way of becoming reassociated with the larger society. As this comes about it will alter existing systems of relations between A-, B-, and C-type centres.

(b) It will entail some sharing of the problems of scientific choice with representatives of the various clienteles with whom social scientists become collaboratively engaged. This will bring into being a new set of criteria for 'co-determination' of research themes and priorities.

(c) The research worker now becomes accountable not only to his scientific colleagues but also to his participating clienteles. This means extending the concept of taking professional responsibility from the service to the research area.

(d) As regards complexity, significant innovations may be expected to arise from group, as distinct from individual, creativeness. This will alter existing systems of status and reward, which have remained individual.

(e) As regards scale, aggregations of resources require to be created so that large-scale problems can be investigated not only with due regard to their scope, which will frequently be transnational, but to their duration, which will frequently transcend the work-life of a given scientific generation.

Reassociating the University with Society

The process of reassociating the university with its larger society is in some respects farther advanced in other parts of the world than in Western Europe. In the United States, universities, especially those which are pre-eminent, have come to be regarded as part of the 'government-industry-education complex'. The implicit disparagement here signals the danger inherent in the reassociation process. Nevertheless, any suggestion that this is merely a temporary aberration shows a lack of understanding of the underlying change. Yet even in the United States there is still no general recognition of problem-oriented research as an inherent strategy for advancing the knowledge base. Nor has enough been done to relate the basic disciplines in comprehensive schools of social sciences. In this last regard some of the most promising developments are those taking place in the newer universities in the United Kingdom.

In the countries of Eastern Europe the split has been between the universities as carriers of the research/teaching mix and the academies of sciences as carriers of the research/application mix. Such a separation represents the type of science policy to be expected in countries requiring simultaneously to develop, from a narrow base, an extensive system of tertiary education and an advanced research capability. The danger of maintaining the separation at the level hitherto obtaining, now that the bases themselves are widening, has been recognized.

In the developing countries the social sciences are perceived as a critical resource for understanding and advancing the process of development. Until recently problems of development had been approached too exclusively in economic and technological terms. Repeated disappointment with the results of programmes of technical and economic aid, and indeed of internally sponsored plans, is creating a new climate. This is characterized by a greater willingness to consider the complex interrelations that exist between cultural, psychological, and social-structural factors and economic and technological aspects. The situation ensuing confronts the social sciences with intensified demands to undertake *actions concertées* – through a route that would give priority first to A-, next to C-, and thence to B-type activities. In the decades ahead the social rather than the natural sciences may take the role of the leading part in the scientific affairs of developing countries.

Joint Responsibility

Questions of sharing scientific choice and taking professional responsibility have been discussed in relation to problems of 'gaining access' to the heavily defended areas of human activity and experience and of working with collaborating clienteles to achieve superordinate goals. Unless this is done matters of central importance to human beings will not be brought to the attention of social scientists, whose researches will be restricted to matters on which little 'value' is placed. For central issues involve questions of values. All questions of social (or personal) change, for example, involve questions of value. The social scientists must either abstain from their study or join with others in their pursuit. They will never be handed over to him for independent experimentation.

Acceptance of joint responsibility by the social scientist and his clienteles is the key. By actively participating in the research effort themselves the representatives of the client systems can allow the social scientist also to take an active role. This may alter the 'appreciation' of the problem. Consequent action decisions remain with the client; consequent implications for theory with the social scientist.

In this model the social scientist takes his place along with the other actors in the starting conditions. By accepting the constraints of being 'included' he gains the requisite degree of freedom to study processes of value-laden social change while they are occurring. If he elects to stay out, he is forced back on retrospective evidence. History by itself is not enough.

Though there are many areas of social science that do not require this strategy, it is not yet realized how many there are that do. The basic organizational form pertinent to this type of study is the jointly engaged group of 'researchers' and 'researched'.

Group Creativeness

That group, in addition to individual, creativeness may be required in face of higher orders of complexity poses organizational problems of a novel character. For the belief is ingrained that scientific innovation is the product of an exceptional but individual mind. The evidence would support this belief, which belongs to the tradition of academic individualism. Yet there is another aspect. Exceptional minds tend to exist in networks of mutual influence extended over space and time. This was so even in the seventeenth and eighteenth centuries, when the natural sciences arose. Under contemporary conditions, these networks have increased in number, in density, in degree of overlap, and in frequency and immediacy of encounter. They represent systems of interpersonal choices in which the individuals concerned become selectively interdependent.[7] Such groups tend to be shifting and temporary. They are rarely bound by formal relations, though their members recognize them as a necessary condition of their capacity to innovate.

The increasing importance of problem-oriented research as a means of advancing fundamental knowledge is strengthening the trend among selectively interdependent groups to form more permanent organizations (i.e. Type C institutes). This arises because problem-oriented research requires operational commitment to a common group task as the means by which a shared direction in scientific ideas can be empirically realized. Since this realization must be accomplished under real-life conditions, relations with various kinds of clienteles are involved. Their trust can be secured only if they experience stability in the research organization.

To achieve this stability such organizations must create a value system based on a co-operative pooling of resources.

(a) This is facilitated by the sharing of a common status among senior members, as by the fellows of a college.
(b) It is reinforced by the experience of group products being superior to individual products.
(c) Yet when some members contribute more than others this requires recognition.
(d) Members of such organizations tend to deploy themselves in loosely coupled overlapping subsets – or assemblies. Recent neurophysiological research has shown that this is how the brain would appear to work (Tomkins, 1964). An analogue of the brain at a higher system level is what one is seeking to discover.

This total configuration is the opposite of academic individualism. It makes a poor match with the fixed roles and statuses of university departments, especially those of the single-professor variety, which this tradition has tended to perpetuate.

In this regard the larger departments common in American universities, with multiple chairs and where associate and assistant professors have a voice in decision-making, afford a better match with what is required. On the other hand, American universities maintain the tradition of academic individualism by forcing the individual scholar to conform to the rule of 'publish or perish'. In the West R & D laboratories in some of the large industrial concerns are organized more in keeping with a group value system than are many universities. Empirical studies are required on what the climate is like and how decisions are made in the institutes of the academies of sciences of Eastern Europe.

In some universities there is a growing tendency not only to form centres of selectively interdependent individuals, drawn from a number of teaching departments, but for these centres to form research consortia with other organizations in different universities and in other countries. Nor are such associations confined to university bodies. The probability is low that the key resources for critical programmes will be found in one place. Nevertheless, these resources need dependable bases if they are to join together in high-risk research expeditions of a temporary, though often protracted, character. An interdependent system of stability and mobility requires to be evolved.

Longitudinal Capability

Another direction of the search for an alternative to academic individualism is the creation of institutional capabilities that would permit the undertaking of large-scale investigations over long periods of time. The basic issue has already been touched on. The increasing rate of change, along with the degree of uncertainty and of environmental complexity characteristic of the contemporary world, is forcing societies to collect more accurate information about their populations, institutions, and individual members, the trends and levels of their economic and social performance, and about other societies. The collection of social and economic facts, however, tends to have been left to governmental bureaucracies which are slow to make use of the latest techniques and resistant to widening categories of information designed to meet limited administrative requirements.

The first problem is to close the gap between existing practice and available concepts and methods. This means either changing the relation between official bodies and sources of social science competence in universities and special institutes or bringing new and more appropriate organizations into existence. While progress is being made in several countries it is too slow to meet society's requirements under conditions of accelerating change.

The second problem concerns the extent to which general-purpose social and economic data are made public. Will they be presented in a form that makes possible independent appraisal by members of the social science community? Only genuine reasons of security should prevent scientifically accountable publication. The obverse of this problem is that concerning the privacy of the individual.

The function of collecting and analysing social and economic data can be most effectively executed and most rapidly developed if made the responsibility of Type C3 and C4 institutes under the control of social scientists appointed by joint agreement between government, universities, and professional associations. Government departments would be the principal, but by no means the only, clienteles of such institutes. They would have their own internal specialists to interpret findings and carry out special purpose analyses. But such institutes would also have the power of initiating inquiries – to assist in building up the corpus of knowledge required to provide a public basis for taking informed social action in all domains of society.

Some of the technical problems in this field are formidable. Data are required over ever-longer periods, but concepts and methods are continuously improving and the foci of investigation continuously shifting. To obtain desired comparisons often proves impossible. A strategically planned attack on such difficulties made on a scientific rather than an administrative basis would obtain solutions improved far beyond what is at present deemed feasible.

One of the most exciting prospects before the social sciences at the present time is the gradual unification of the disciplines depending on historical and on contemporary sources of evidence. Improved collection of basic social and economic data is the best method of obtaining what might be termed the extension of the present. The more man must prepare to meet an uncertain future and to construct alternative models of what that future might be, the greater is his need for information that will yield an extension of the present.

Here the continuing development of computer technology for the organization of large-scale files of mass data for quick retrieval and analysis is bound to prove of decisive importance. The organization of data archives for historical as well as contemporary information will change fundamentally the conditions for cumulative collective research in the social sciences: data archives will not only create a broader basis for collective efforts of analysis, interpretation, and the planning of fresh research, but will also ensure linkage over time from one project to another, since the results of new analysis will be incorporated with the old information in the machine-accessible storage media. The data archives will add a new dimension to the social science libraries and will change the character of social science teaching and training (Rokkan, 1966).

Notes

[1] For the concept of directive correlation see Sommerhof (1950).

[2] An illuminating (and amusing) example is given by Price (1965, op. cit.) in his account of the struggle of oceanography to find a place in the federal scientific system of the United States.

[3] This scheme is developed from *Social Research and a National Policy for Science* (Tavistock Institute of Human Relations, 1964).

[4] This Committee was set up by the Committee on Science and Public Policy of the National Academy of Sciences and the Problems and Policy Committee of the Social Science Research Council in the United States (National Research Council/Social Science Research Council, 1969).

[5] For the report of the policy statement issued see UNESCO, 1970.

[6] For an account of the development of the concept of the leading part in biology and its extension to the social sciences see Andras Angyal (1958).

[7] This term is due to F. E. Emery.

References

ACKOFF, R. L., Games, Decisions and Organisations. *General Systems Yearbook*, Ann Arbor, Michigan, 1959.

ANGYAL, ANDRAS, *Foundations for a Science of Personality*. Harvard University Press, Cambridge, Mass., 1958.

ASHBY, R., General Systems as a New Discipline. *General Systems Yearbook*, Ann Arbor, Michigan, 1959.

BELL, D., Twelve Modes of Prediction. *Survey of the Social Sciences*, Penguin, Harmondsworth, 1964.

— (ed.), The Year 2000: the Trajectory of an Idea, *Daedalus* **96**, 3, 1967.

BIE, PIERRE DE, Introduction to Special Issue on Multidisciplinary Problem-focused Research. *International Social Science Journal* **20**, 2, 1968.

BRIM, O., Statement at ISSC Conference on Social Science Policy. Paris, 1970.

CHERNS, A. B., Relations between Research Institutions and Users of Research. *International Social Science Journal* **22**, 2, pp. 226–42, 1970.

CHEVALIER, M., Stimulation of Needed Social Science Research for Canadian Water Resource Problems. Privy Council Science Secretariat, Queen's Printer, Ottawa, 1967.

CHURCHMAN, W. C., *et al.*, *Experiments on Enquiring Systems*. Report of the Social Sciences Group, Space Sciences Laboratory, University of California, Berkeley, 1967.

EMERY, F. E., The Next Thirty Years: Concepts, Methods, and Anticipations. *Human Relations* **20**, 3, pp. 199–237, 1967.

EMERY, F. E. and THORSRUD, E., *Form and Content in Industrial Democracy.* Tavistock Publications, London, 1969.
ERICKSON, J., Statement at Edinburgh Conference on the Impact of Science and Technology, 1970.
GROSS, B., *The State of the Nation.* Tavistock Publications, London, 1966.
KAPLAN, A., *The Conduct of Inquiry.* Chandler, San Francisco, 1964.
LAWRENCE, J. R. (ed.), *Operational Research and the Social Sciences.* Tavistock Publications, London, 1964.
MCWHINNEY, W., Organisational Form, Decision Modalities, and the Environment. *Human Relations* **21**, 3, pp. 269–81, 1968.
MEDAWAR, SIR PETER, *The Art of the Soluble.* Methuen, London, 1967.
National Research Council/Social Science Research Council, *The Behavioral and Social Sciences: Outlook and Needs.* Prentice-Hall, Englewood Cliffs, N.J., 1969.
PARSONS, T., *Structure and Process in Modern Societies.* Free Press, Glencoe, 1960.
PERLMUTTER, H. V., *Towards a Theory and Practice of Social Architecture.* Tavistock Publications, London, 1965.
POLANYI, M., The Growth of Science in Society. *Minerva* **5**, 4, pp. 533–45, 1967.
PRICE, D. K., *The Scientific Estate.* Belknap, Cambridge, Mass., 1965.
REES, J. R., *The Shaping of Psychiatry by War.* Norton, New York, 1945.
ROKKAN, S. (ed.), *Data Archives in the Social Sciences.* Mouton, Paris, 1966.
SANFORD, N., *General Education and Research on Human Problems.* Institute for the Study of Human Problems, Stanford, 1963.
SOMMERHOF, G., *Analytical Biology.* Oxford University Press, London. 1950.
Tavistock Institute of Human Relations (Council), *Social Research and a National Policy for Science.* Tavistock Publications, London, 1964.
TOMKINS, S., *Affect, Imagery and Consciousness,* Vol. 1. Springer, New York, 1964.
TRIST, E. L., *The Relation of Welfare and Development in the Transition to Post-Industrialism,* Canadian Centre for Community Studies, Ottawa, 1967.
— Organization and Financing of Social Science Research. In *The Main Trends of Research in the Social and Human Sciences.* UNESCO, Mouton, Paris, 1970.
— HIGGIN, G. W., MURRAY, H., POLLOCK, A. B., *Organizational Choice: Capabilities of Groups at the Coal Face under Changing Technologies.* Tavistock Publications, London, 1963.
— and SOFER, C., *Explorations in Group Relations.* Leicester University Press, Leicester, 1959.
UNESCO, Science Policy Division, *National Science Policies of the United States: Origins, Development and Present Status.* UNESCO, Paris, 1968.
UNESCO, International Co-operation on the Development of Social Science Research. Report of a Round Table on Social Research Policy and Organization. *International Social Science Journal* **22**, 1, 1970.
United Nations, *Appraising Administrative Capability for Development.* UN, New York, 1969.
VICKERS, SIR GEOFFREY, *The Art of Judgement.* Chapman & Hall, London, 1965.
— *Value Systems and Social Process.* Tavistock Publications, London, 1968.
— *Freedom in a Rocking Boat.* Allen Lane, The Penguin Press, London, 1970.

Interchapter

We discussed the problems of research institutes in the social sciences – where should they be, what 'mix' should they provide, what issues should they tackle? Should research institutes be located within the university system? Eric Trist emphasized that there is no clear answer, since location depends on context. He has had experience of institutes, both separate from and integrated with universities; many problems of the latter demonstrated the need to change university values, not only towards approval for contract research, but also towards returning overheads on research contracts to the institute to sustain its growth. Without these inputs, groups cannot fund themselves for exploratory work, for supporting their graduate students between contracts, or even for writing research proposals. Another issue facing institutes within American universities is the need to unite the concept of faculty with the concept of research staff. Tenure is important and in many cases has been denied professional research workers. In some instances this leads to institutes being removed from university contexts. The research-teaching link has to be defined in such a way that the institute member can spend a good proportion of time in the research centre and have students working on field projects. Institutes, when closely linked to academic structures, admittedly run the risk of becoming discipline bound and hence unable to innovate and change with the times. The University of Michigan's Institute for Social Research has learned how to add new centres to itself and to set up inter-centre programmes, and this is a move in the right direction.

Stein Rokkan agreed with Eric Trist. Michigan has flexible arrangements between departments and the Institute with regard to tenure and institute-departmental mobility. However, these arrangements are generally restricted to senior workers. The Institute for Social Research has been able to retain a large proportion of overheads through an arrangement negotiated on the Institute's establishment.

Returning to the more general points involving institute location, Professor Wilson drew attention to the nature and significance of academic individualism. This characteristic is built into university life and would drive research institutes outside the university system, minimizing the possibility of collaborative research. Drawing upon the German experience, Dietrich Goldschmidt sees the causes of individualism as deep-rooted, both in the social norms of the scientific enterprise and the substantive nature of the problem that was being investigated and also in factors such as the logistics of the present situation, where low teacher–student ratios (1 : 20) leave little opportunity for collaborative work. New universities developed in post-war Germany have, in part at least, been designed to overcome some of these problems. However, these have perpetuated individualistic efforts rather than opposed them. The older generation of academics has been socialized too thoroughly for established habits to be broken. Thus institutes independent of universities have arisen chiefly out of the failures of the university, which must seek a more effective remedy than seemed currently available, particularly as it continues to lose high level manpower. Yet, to achieve this, as another participant was quick to point out, involves recognizing the internal disjunction between administrative policies and reward systems. Thus, in the US, individual publications in pure research are frequently supported, while the institution has committed itself to problem-based interdisciplinary programmes. Such programmes struggle to progress in the face of a lack of support from academics in disciplinary departments who see in these efforts little opportunity for new kinds of work.

To Henning Friis, however, the argument for linking research institutes closely to universities was not as attractive as to some of the other participants, particularly where applied social research was concerned. Some years earlier, Professor Friis was attracted to the ideas sponsored by the Tavistock Institute (UK) of initiating domain-based problem research institutes, both inside and outside universities. However, his opinion now is that policy-makers should not expect universities to take on applied research. Universities could attempt such tasks but at the considerable risk that not only would their speed of working be too slow (from the policy-makers' viewpoint) but they might digress on a tangent induced by the lure of fundamental research. As a consequence, the results they produced would not be relevant even for long-range policy issues. Applied social research should therefore be undertaken in strong self-sustaining institutes outside universities. This did not argue against institutes within university structures, but these should concentrate on fundamental work.

Replying to some of the comments made, Professor Trist first took up the point of whether domain-based problem-oriented research should be based within the universities. We must take into account indications that in many areas theories and concepts are not advanced enough to provide internally generated problems. In some areas of economics theory leads the way, but this does not seem the case for most areas of the social sciences. Field determination of problems allows the researcher to respond to the demand and texture of his society. In different societies, at different moments of history, different opportunities are offered for problem solution and theoretical advance, linked however to the state of the relevant disciplines. This work is feasible both inside and outside university structures. In answer to a query of whether externally based applied research too easily slips into consultancy, Trist acknowledged this as a problem that exists and has to be faced. Frequently when one takes up a project opportunity, one does not know what it is going to turn into. In brief, the research is not predetermined. Only after working on the problem for some substantial time can one be sure that there is something of social science significance there. If not, one must have the means to withdraw from or to terminate the project, since it is not practical to use up resources on service-type arrangements. Even enterprises that from the outside seem ambitious programmes may internally have become completely conventionalized.

In conclusion, Professor Trist touched on the topic of institutional size. Within universities a unit can exist on a much smaller scale than if it were independent. Independent institutions seem, in the long run, unable to survive with fewer than 30 to 35 scientific staff. The dilemma is that this increased size brings problems of bureaucratization, while small units battle against the dangers of instability and low commitment of staff. In general, as well as a base organization, one needs connections with other institutes. It is essential to develop systems and networks within countries and across countries. Increasingly flourishing research institutes appear to have developed a network character but a strong institutional base is needed to provide the flexibility to do this.

7 For a school of application of social sciences

Henri Mendras

The changing nature of activities being conducted within both public and private sectors, together with the widening scope of the problems these sectors deal with, precipitate situations that demand the knowledge and experience that can be offered through social science disciplines. These disciplines, however, have developed in such a manner that they provide no 'visible technology'. Application of social science knowledge is much discussed but little practised, while the social engineer or 'applied social scientist' remains an elusive being. Application is a concept that is rarely well received by established university-based social scientists; yet demands for more formal institutional structures through which social science application can be both taught and practised have been a feature of several recent national moves in the the social science policy area.

The French educational system is perhaps more influenced by tradition and long-established institutional systems than any other in Europe. The establishment of innovatory programmes within it poses formal problems. In this chapter[1] Henri Mendras discusses possible means of overcoming these problems, particularly as regards establishing an institutional capacity to produce applied social scientists. The need for such men in both public life and the private sector can already be seen, and their absence is causing identifiable difficulties. Mendras argues that the training of such men can be achieved within the present system and outlines the type of training that should be undertaken.

Henri Mendras is Professor of Sociology at the Centre for Sociological Studies at the University of Nanterre. His past work has been concerned with rural sociology and with the development of programmes for teaching social science to business professionals. His publications include: *Les Paysans dans la France contemporaine* (with Jean Fauvet, 1958) and *Sociologie de la campagne française* (1959).

If history and law were the main sciences of the nineteenth century, sociology, psychology, and economics are certainly those of the twentieth century.

Thanks to its psychometric techniques, psychology has crept into the life of all business enterprises and into the army, the largest of them all. Social psychology has improved amazingly in recent years; the use of opinion polls is becoming a common technique in government. Every industrial man when launching a product, appeals to market research and motivation studies; elections are prepared with similar methods.

For fifteen years, long- and short-term economic programming has become customary in industry as well as in politics. Conjectural policy is becoming more and more efficient. American prosperity, the German miracle, French-style planning, these successes would have been impossible without the intervention of economic science, whatever may be the doctrines propounded by governments. It is therefore logical that the teaching of economics should have its place in the Institut d'Études politiques and École nationale d'administration, just as in the schools of engineering. Similarly, the parts of administration and private companies whose power increases are economic entities.

On the contrary, sociology is a younger discipline, less sure of its instruments of analysis and intervention. Certain people expect that it should resolve all the problems left behind by the economists; others say it is useless and see it only as a new ideology. Taken as an isolated discipline it deserves neither so much trust nor so much concern. Above all, and this fact is quite new, it is bound up with social psychology and economics, and constitutes a body of knowledge, resting on an intellectual process common to all the social sciences. Nowadays, the teaching of sociology is almost totally separate from that of economics. For the students it is hard to understand that what they are taught in the Faculty of Law is the same as what they are made to learn in the Faculty of Arts: it is a means to master the evolution of economic and social life by understanding it.

Personally I believe in the existence of a social science that is a rigorous intellectual discipline capable of moulding young brains, a tool of analysis and intervention adapted to post-industrial society. Besides which it might breed a new culture, lead to a new humanism, and play in the twentieth century the traditional role of arts, philosophy, history, and law in the production of an educated gentleman. In fact it gives the sense of relativity that formerly one acquired by reading the great classics. On the other hand, economic and sociological analysis performed according to the strict rules of logic is an exercise of intellectual rigour that can replace the Latin Version and the Commentary of Jurisdiction.

This claim may appear extreme and this is not the place to discuss it; however, I believe it to be well founded. If it is so, and if the evolution of society leads to a greater consistency between science and social action, it is of paramount importance to form a clear idea of the different types of competence that are going to become essential for the proper functioning of our society, to imagine the careers that will offer themselves tomorrow to young people, and, most important of all, to create institutions to train young people for these careers.

NEW CAREERS IN PUBLIC LIFE

The proliferation of consultancies and advisory bodies to which both government and business have recourse shows that the need for applied social science is felt throughout, but that existing institutions do not know how to respond to it by their own means. Undoubtedly the public services have been more progressive in this respect than industry. The 'Commissariat au Plan' of the Forties and Fifties remains the principal concern of the consultant bodies, imitated in many fields and in many countries. A group of experts in social science called together by virtue of their capabilities and with the aim of fixing the objectives of action for external authorities which are jealous of their prerogatives – isn't this the definition of all planning services, national, international, regional, and industrial?

In Bobodioulasso, Brussels, or Detroit, as well as in Moscow and Havana, the model invented by Jean Monnet multiplies, proliferates, and adapts itself to greatly differing situations and conditions. The people who compose such organizations consider themselves experts, some would say technocrats. Their professional position is defined neither by belonging to an organization, nor by their dependence on a political clientele, nor by their hierarchical position. Usually, they are neither civil servants nor politicians delegated to the supervision of a mechanism of power, nor managers responsible for their decisions. They do, however, perform tasks that were generally entrusted to a minister's advisers and they command a great deal of power because they prepare, and therefore orientate, the decisions of a great number of politicians and businessmen.

To improve the administrative structure of the nineteenth century, a large body of national and regional planning engineers should be created. This body would be a source of inspiration and information to the experts and would be sent to various organizations, to the European community in Brussels, to the planning service of an African, a South American, or an Asian capital, but would also take part in all enterprises of regional or community development. Besides, a great number of these technocrats would be content to quit the civil service and use their skills in the service of big business, which would procure their collaboration at a high price.

Such is the French way of creating a career and an *esprit de corps,* which would be smashed almost as soon as it was formed. The Anglo-Saxon way of doing things would be to set up an old-school-tie network of individuals following careers, as socioeconomic experts or as engineers in social science in big firms, who from time to time would join the civil service or travel to foreign countries as advisers, before succumbing to the temptation of a university chair.

NEW CAREERS IN THE PRIVATE SECTOR

This sketch gives an outline picture of public and semi-public careers which could be extended and staffed with competent personnel. But in which careers in the private sector could the same skills be used? – in employment departments and public relations.

In many large American companies, social relations are entrusted to a vice-president; in the large French firms this responsibility is most often entrusted to people who have not succeeded elsewhere, in the technical and commercial departments. As one of the most brilliant and successful human relations specialists said in jest: the profession doesn't exist, and in so far as it does it is staffed by failures. It is evident that for this profession, which should offer a brilliant and fascinating career, it is impossible today to propose a specialized course of training or education to any young person who feels he has a vocation for such a career; if he were to follow in his predecessors' steps any form of higher education would be equally recommendable.

Fixing social policy within a business firm, negotiating a collective agreement with trade unions, modifying a system of remuneration, remodelling a hierarchical structure, fixing recruitment criteria, predicting human problems presented by an amalgamation of businesses or by the transfer of a factory from one region to another, organizing refresher courses for managers and tradesmen – these tasks, in a business where personnel expenditure can represent 60 per cent of turnover, demand skills that cannot be improvised. It is not sufficient to have tact and initiative and the capacity to command authority. Traditionally in a factory the personnel manager could be an officer quite separate from the managers, because his role was mainly to supervise discipline, to administer, and to settle legal difficulties. But in a firm that has numerous establishments and whose administrative services are as important as the productive ones, the person in charge of social relations should have an economics and sociology training and should know how to use the techniques of intervention of the psycho-sociologist. According to an inquiry of the National Association of Personnel Directors and Managers (ANDCP), 60 per cent of their members consider that the human sciences should occupy first place in the curriculum for training their young colleagues.[2] Moreover they all insist on the human qualities, the character and personality that the job demands, but they agree in thinking that these qualities are developed and made more efficient by psychological, economic, and sociological knowledge.

A similar inquiry conducted by AFAP among people responsible for external communications in businesses reveals more definite opinions. Some older lorry-drivers declared abruptly: 'I cannot understand that they come to give lessons in psychology to people who have practised their profession for twenty-five or thirty years.' For them, in fact, the 'psychological qualities' are no different from knowledge accumulated by scientific psychology (AFAP, 1967). Opposing this idea is an avant-garde group, which finds its recruits particularly among those responsible for publicity and considers that a general education in social sciences is necessary in order to understand the reactions of men from different social categories and to determine the form and basis of messages addressed to the consumers.

In as far as one can no longer be content to sell what one produces but must produce what one can sell, the traditional commercial department is replaced by a group of more complex services with various names: sales promotion, market research, marketing, public relations, publicity. The ensemble that these services make up is charged with co-ordinating the external relations of the business and at the same time to create in public opinion a favourable attitude to the name of the firm, make products known to the public, and pass on necessary information to the commercial network. Economic and sociological intelligence should be amassed and organized so as to serve to define the policy of the firm: once this has been fixed it should be passed on to the advertising departments and to the commercial network. The task of co-ordinating and orientating these functions can no longer be done with just experience, business sense, and dynamism: knowledge of the social sciences and of techniques is essential to everyday operation.

In his preface to Katchourine's book, Jean Stoetzel is right to insist on 'the general mistrust felt by practical people for with respect to scientific people: that, for example, of the small industrial contractor, still quite prevalent at the beginning of the century, towards the engineer coming out of the university, that of the peasant towards the agronomist, or, furthermore, that of the political expert towards opinion polls. One must fully understand this mistrust' (Katchourine, 1967) which is not always a more serious difficulty in the dialogue between the social scientist and the practical man than is the exaggerated confidence some people show in the magic of science, from which they expect recipes that it cannot provide. Katchourine concludes that 'the place accorded to the human sciences in the field of public relations is still quite limited in the minds of the great majority of those questioned; these people are trying above all to obtain ways of influencing the public from the human sciences'. On the contrary, 'advertising executives' consider that 'the interest of the human sciences exceeds that of the acquisition of certain techniques, for a psycho-social culture opens the mind and affords a new understanding of beings and things'. Anyway, all agree that 'a reform of the teaching of human sciences is indispensable. There is no unified scheme of teaching these sciences and each is taught in a too formal and insufficient style' (Katchourine, 1967).

The meetings organized periodically by the Royaumont Foundation between sociologists, business-owners, and managing directors of large firms have clearly brought to light the eagerness to gain some knowledge of sociology as well as the difficulty of dialogue. During one of these meetings, Raymond Barre underlined the necessity for creating a new profession, that of business sociologist, rather like the business economist who has multiplied in the last decade.

Industrial managements should include sociological advisers if they wish to be able to use the services of advertising agents and organizational consultants with discrimination. 'The main agencies deplore the lack of capable experts with whom to liaise. Often the client has neither the time nor sufficient competence to use the results of their work correctly. They prefer to work for firms which have their own properly organized market research department who, even though they are more demanding, appreciate the quality of their work and know how to exploit the results' (Katchourine, 1967). In the United States the big companies that call in sociologists regularly are those that have within their own management sociologists of international standing who have been university professors and who often become professors again afterwards. The dialogue between the practical men and the researcher is never easy and the need for a third person is felt by both parties for reasons meriting detailed analysis, which I have sketched out elsewhere (Mendras, 1963; Lazarsfeld *et al.*, 1967).

Finally, there exists another career, almost non-existent at the present time in France, that of research administrator – whether it stems from the public or private sector one does not know. In the university, in large research bodies, and in the largest firms, it is necessary to run more and more numerous and expensive laboratories, and the traditional rules of industrial management, which measures its results by its profits, and of university administration, which measures its success by the prestige of its experts, are no longer sufficient. One must compound these two pictures in order to make decisions and to allocate enormous resources to businesses in jeopardy. Consequently one must organize the functioning of these huge research enterprises whether they are private or public companies. The United States drains away the best European brains simply by offering them better working conditions, hence the high percentage of Nobel Prizes awarded to the USA, which scandalizes Europe. How are we to train the administrators of our universities, of the National Scientific Research Centre, and of the industrial research organizations?

Is it arbitrary to include under the same rubric careers as different as those just enumerated, to which one would undoubtedly have to add several others? I don't think so, for they have certain characteristics and demands in common. They require a certain understanding of the functioning of widely differing societies and of the contribution the social sciences can make towards it; on the other hand these careers have an advisory nature rather than that of decision-making or policy execution. If its outlets are so numerous, what should be the recruitment and teaching programme of this school of application of the social sciences?

TEACHING PROGRAMME

Let us imagine that each year in France one hundred or so social science engineers have to be trained. The most effective way of doing this in the present state of our educational system would be to attract former pupils of the 'Grandes écoles' (Polytechnique centrale, etc.), people with degrees in sociology, economics, psychology, and political science. No age limit would be imposed. The choice of candidates would be at the discretion of a selection commission, as is the case both at the CEPE and for admission to the second year of the Institute of Political Studies. The candidate would submit a written composition on a general subject and be interviewed by the commission. A ruling would be given on the basis of university file, past professional record, written composition, and interview.

The course of study would last two years. The teaching would cover three principal areas: economics, sociology, and methods (logic and mathematics). During the first year, the teachers would aim to bring students from widely differing origins to a common level. The engineers would be taught economics and, above all, sociology; the economists would be taught sociology and methods; the sociologists and psychologists would study mainly economics and methods. All would be obliged to undertake a practical course in English with the aid of audio-visual techniques, and almost all would have to do editorial exercises and public speaking: to know how to organize one's ideas and to express them clearly by writing or speaking in English and French is a capacity required by all the careers envisaged above. Even graduates do not always possess these abilities any more. During the second year, teaching will include one part common to all students and various special subjects.

In the course of the two years, formal lecturing would be limited to the main technical matters, which demand an ordered exposition, and to 'information' matters composed of balanced descriptions and subtle analyses. This formal teaching would aim not only to pass on knowledge but also to provide some material for synthetic lectures and discussions.

The greater part of the time would be devoted to seminars and small group teaching, both as individuals and in groups, to discussions, and to a practical introduction to the different techniques of the social sciences. Since one wishes to train neither cabinet economists nor theoretical sociologists but social science engineers, one would attach little importance to the theory of each of these disciplines and would insist upon the connections between analysis, method, technique, and 'reality'. If I dare say so, essentially this teaching should be centred on practical epistemology and contribute to a science of the application of science.

In economics less place would be given to theory than to economic politics. Economics would be concerned with a practical initiation to the functioning of the national economy and industrial life: the state's instruments of intervention, financial and banking procedures, techniques of business management, national and management accounting, different forms of planning, etc. An important place would be given to rural economies, to the problems of industrialization of underdeveloped countries, to international commerce, and to the economic policies of various countries. To give the students a sense of the breadth of the problems and of the chronology of events, geography and economic history would be part of the curriculum. One would strongly emphasize the theoretical nature of the models and would put the students on their guard against the pitfalls of confusing concepts and reality, e.g. the young economist who believes that the Gross National Product is something that exists.

This precaution is equally important in sociology: one would wish to point out that notions explain reality but do not describe it. One expects that sociology will challenge the reassuring rationality of the economist and reintroduce the notions of value and the sense of relativity. Sociological theory will be restricted to those theories on which all sociologists agree, and quarrels between different schools of thought would only be introduced in so far as they exemplify epistemological problems. Ethnology and social history will have a place in describing the variety of social systems and the evolution of events, for example the history of the trade union movement and labour relations, and, of course, political history would be taught in conjunction with industrial and political sociology. Furthermore, the study of experiments in social psychology (communications, small groups, sociometry, etc.) would be included also.

The methodological part would comprise logic, mathematics, and methodology (variables, plans of analysis, indicators, indices, etc.). To show to what extent economic and sociological analysis is bound up with its techniques of investigation, one must introduce the students to the practical handling of these techniques: statistics, accounting, drawing up questionnaires, procedures of inquiry (interviews, etc.), coding, eliciting information, interpretation. Finally, an introduction to the use of computers and machine languages would complete this third part, which would also afford a glimpse into the modern methods of arriving at a decision, theory of games, simulation.

In addition to these three fundamental sectors, languages and rhetoric would have their place, and undoubtedly a minimum of legal theory (public law, private law, labour law) would have to be taught.

This programme may appear enormous: it would be if it was intended for young people without any previous training, but each student would already have a serious training in one of the three basic sectors and a habit of personal study. The recruitment of the teaching body, the creation of a fruitful teacher–pupil relationship, the use of modern teaching techniques and the progressive disposition of the programme would undoubtedly present the most delicate problems. University men, researchers, and technicians would join a group teaching full time, which would include supervision and a number of professors responsible for the main disciplines. For economics, pedagogic techniques exist; for sociology, they are in process of development;[3] and for methods and techniques, materials already exist. But one would have to put on a proper footing a whole battery of new instruments: practical projects, case studies, files to prepare, inquiries to develop and interpret, etc.

ANCILLARY INSTITUTIONS

Once the programme and methods have been settled, it would be easy to transpose them into two types of different institution. For men already occupying positions in business or in the public services one could organize teaching of an evening-class type, similar to what has been done at the Centre of Preparation for Business (CPA) of the Paris Chamber of Commerce or, in a different style, at the Research Centre of Business Directors (CRC) of the CNPF (National Council of Business Management). For people having practical experience, the programme could be lightened and specialized in various sections corresponding to their careers. One might also contemplate giving them scholarships to enable them to follow the normal courses at the school for two years. On the other hand, if one wanted to train a body of middle managers corresponding to the upper elite trained by the school, one might envisage the development of university institutes of technology. The best students of these could have access to the school.

On leaving our main institutions of higher education (École normale or École des Chartes), some students go abroad to the École de Rome, the École d'Athènes or la Casa Velasquez. One could imagine in the same manner 'French schools of economics and sociology' in certain countries, either 'highly developed' countries (for example, at Princeton, Harvard, Oxford, Moscow, or Novosibirsk), where students would go to perfect their studies or to specialize in a particular sector, or 'underdeveloped' countries, where students could study problems of development. In both cases they would come back with a thesis and take a research doctorate. A prolonged stay in a foreign country is essential in the training of social science specialists who need time to get to know a country (and its language) and who possess their discipline as a craftsman possesses his tools for only in applying it to a foreign society can they place themselves at a distance when looking at their own society. One needs to create some 'Villa Medicis' for the social sciences. Let us imagine the House of Gobineau in Teheran transformed into a 'Maison française des sciences sociales'. Each year one could offer a scholarship for two years to former pupils of the school to which might come a geographer, an economist, a sociologist, an ethnologist, young researchers, or future professors. Are the advantages of such an institution immediately clear? Researchers, university people, and social science engineers would learn to get to know each other and argue their points of view.

Young foreign experts completing their training would do basic research in the logic of underlying scientific principles, and would not be restricted to answering the local politicians' questions. But, not being able to escape that country's problems, they would feel themselves obliged to answer them. And, in social science, the best applied research is that which poses theoretical problems in connection with social issues. We would have a mass of comparative research, which would contribute to the theory of economic development and social change.

Notes

[1] Revised version of a paper published in *Analyse et Prévision* 5, May, 1968.

[2] Information provided by M. Toupet, President of ANDCP, and others, whom I thank warmly.

[3] Further to the collections of PUF and Plon, a collection of elementary manuals is in preparation by A. Colin (the first volume has just come out: H. Mendras, *Éléments de sociologie:* and a selection of more advanced readers is about to be published by Mouton.

References

AFAP, Service de Psychologie Appliqué, Les Communications extérieures de l'entreprise, September 1967, Ronéo.

KATCHOURINE, ALEC, *La Psychologie sociale clé du marketing apport de la psychologie sociale aux communications commerciales.* SABRI, Paris, 1967.

LAZARSFELD, PAUL, *et al., The Uses of Sociology.* Basic Books, New York, 1967.

MENDRAS, H., *Sociologie de la campagne française.* Presses Universitaires de France, Paris, 1959.

— Du Diagnostic et de l'ordonnance thérapeutique en sociologie. *Revue française de Sociologie*, No. 4, pp. 433–44, 1963.

MENDRAS, H., and FAUVET, J., *Les Paysans dans la France contemporaine.* Paris, 1958.

Interchapter

The influence of ideology on patterns of utilization was one major theme of the discussions on Henri Mendras's paper. Mendras moved out from the specific topic of his paper to reflect on the successes and failures of the social sciences in French society. The two main areas where the social sciences are really used in France are by the Catholic Church and in the establishment and refinement of opinion polls. In the Fifth Republic the opinion poll became a tool of government. Can we then evaluate its influence on governmental decisions and on the public itself? A project to study these influences would provide an interesting case history on the relationship between social science, society, and decision-making.

The Catholic Church however provides the best success story of social science in France. In terms of money, or of numbers of people involved, social science has been extensively used by the Church for over twenty years. The initiatives often lay with the priests themselves, and there now exists a census of religious practice for almost every French parish. These provide indicators of religious life, which act as the basis for comparisons between religious practice and other statistical indicators. Perhaps even more important is the fact that sociology is now used to manage the Church, and to change its ideology and practice. In almost every diocese there is now at least one priest who is a sociologist; and ecclesiastical missions are only carried out after social surveys of the districts in question. This illustration of the use of sociology by an enormous organization, together with its use in refining opinion polls, constitute two important examples of successful utilization.

A third example, continued Mendras, is provided by the activities of Michel Crozier, who, following the publication of his book *The Bureaucratic Phenomenon*, formed a large group of workers round him and is now probably leading the largest team for sociological research in Paris. His book had a significant impact on French administrators. Indeed, the new Fifth Republic was to a great extent inspired by M. Crozier. How did this come about? In part through ideology, and particularly because many advisers to the French Government were former pupils of Crozier. Hence, considering the three examples together, it would appear that the impact of sociology in France on matters such as governmental doctrine or university reform was through ideology. The major problem of utilization is therefore not influence (as suggested by Dr Crawford) but ideology, and social science will only succeed when it becomes ideology. Economics succeeded by giving policy-makers an economic ideology and enabling them to see society through an economist's eyes. The other social sciences have made only limited progress towards this goal.

Taking up Mendras's final point, Cherns was interested in this apparent success of the French sociologists in penetrating areas where ideology was action. He has frequently underlined the importance of directing research into action channels in order that it can be used, and, although it may be stating a tautology, it appears that if sociologists are generating inputs into ideology, the only area where they are likely to be used is the ideological arena. Because of a sociological tradition in France that is ideological rather than empirical, French sociologists have generated inputs into ideological action channels (e.g. opinion polls and economics) rather than supplying engineering solutions in such fields as urban and rural sociology. However, Cherns continued, there is little evidence to show that sociologists (other than a very small minority) in any cultural context have contributed the type of engineering solutions that users normally want, rather they have succeeded in penetrating structures of ideas and modifying them slightly. This process is longer and more arduous than that described by Professor Mendras. The best example in the UK is the influence of sociology on education. Yet some see this as neither good sociology nor good ideology! In the specific case of economics, its practitioners had managed to identify and analyse problems by adopting the mythology of the policy-maker. Sociology, psychology, and political science need to be able to analyse ongoing situations in ways that are as familiar and useful to the policy sector as those provided by economics. To say that economists had the ear of policy-makers because they had usable information perpetuates the idea that all economic data are in fact usable and this is part of the mythology and ideology that the other social sciences are up against.

Further support for Mendras was provided by Orville Brim, with examples from the US. A brief examination of the American policy and advisory structures shows social scientists in positions of some apparent influence. They are in the White House, and they are on prestigeful committees, such as the Council for Economic Advisors. Yet, although so close to the making of policy, their ideologies frequently differ from those of the politicians and administrators. On a more general level, psychologists and sociologists in the US, unlike economists, nearly always differ ideologically from the federal government, although how this relates to the relative successes and failures of social science is not immediately clear.

Replying, Henri Mendras said he was not putting forward the view that French sociology is generally ideologically oriented. Much of the work indeed is empirical; however, the relation between the politician or the higher civil servant and the sociologist is an ideological relationship since French decision-makers use economics as an ideology and they therefore expect the same from sociology. This meant that the relationship between the sociologist and the decision-maker had to be an ideological one. When referring to economics, he had in mind principally that part of the discipline typified by the public accounting taught to higher civil servants. Significantly, many French schools of public administration, which twenty years ago taught general social studies, now devote themselves almost entirely to courses of vulgarized economics. The spread of this way of thinking into government partly explains its affection for public opinion polls. Recent changes in the administrative structure of the French government opened it to greater penetration by economists and such changes seem frequently to bear no relation to the actual life of the people as reflected by social changes in France. Thus, the Ministry of Public Culture, which twenty years ago had been a social and political ministry, was now in composition and thought an economic ministry, although paradoxically the problems it dealt with remained social rather than economic.

On the more general topic of successes and failures in the application of research, Professor Carvalho discussed the difficulties of applying social science in Brazil. Changes in the social structure are needed, but factors such as local government and constitutional elements are difficult to alter. The one hope is incremental change involving neutral modifications of society – neutral at least from the policy-maker's viewpoint. Meetings now being initiated between representatives of government and social science may lead to more effective applications than have been achieved to date: previous suggestions for minor societal changes (arising from the evidence of research projects) have been rejected by the political leadership.

In conclusion, Dr Brim thought that the cases quoted by Professor Mendras illustrated the complexities of studying successful or unsuccessful utilization. Although some insights may be gained from crossnational comparative case studies (as suggested by other conference participants) considerable attention must first be given to questions of differential success within individual countries. During the conference he had picked out from the discussions examples of occasions where the influence of social science on public policy seemed to have been successful, and it would appear that each example bore only a passing relationship to any of the others. So many variables enter into each case that the major initial task was to unravel and identify them.

Agreeing with Brim, Andrew Shonfield noted a shift in the discussions from talking generally about the social sciences to a specific consideration of sociology. This neglects the development of the different disciplines within the same cultural context; in Britain, for example, there is increased use of economists in government as compared to sociologists. We therefore need to examine more carefully the differential uses of disciplines within individual countries and even further we must identify what 'bits' of a discipline are being used. It is, of course, interesting to see whether sociologists are employed or used, but more to the point it is necessary to see what aspects of sociological thinking have penetrated into the decision-making process.

Reference

CROZIER, MICHEL, *Le Phénomène bureaucratique*. Éditions du Seuil, Paris, 1963; *The Bureaucratique Phenomen*. Tavistock Publications, London, 1964.

8 The state of the social sciences

A Round Table Discussion on R & D statistics

Policies for the social sciences, for the continuing support, diversification, and expansion of ongoing activities, require first and foremost to be founded on a knowledge base of what resources currently exist. Unfortunately, at both national and international level, this situation is far from clear. Little is known of the state of the social sciences, as regards either their present condition or the circumstances surrounding the disciplines' development. The demand for information on the social sciences, especially as regards the distribution of money and manpower, is becoming increasingly acute from a political viewpoint. Social scientists themselves, however, are also becoming more interested in the state of their disciplines, although their concerns are frequently of a more theoretical nature.

Such a meeting of interests, in part reinforcing, in part conflicting, underlies current concerns with the collection and collation of statistics on social science activities. In this chapter, some of the past history of efforts in this area is discussed, together with some of the difficulties of pursuing activities of this nature. The chapter also contains an account of a Round Table Discussion on this topic which took place at the Paris Conference; here social scientists and administrators examine how activities in this area might be developed and attempt to identify aspects of such activities where administrative and scientific interests might conflict.

INTRODUCTION

Contemporary studies in the social sciences have focused on a wide variety of processes and structures both within and across cultures. Such activities have tended, perhaps predictably, to become concentrated on certain problem areas rather than being evenly spread across a wide spectrum. Yet paradoxically one sector that has escaped with little attention is the social organization of the social sciences themselves. This reluctance to embark on a process of analytical narcissism may well be understandable; however, it has resulted in the situation where the social scientist, while claiming a patchy but perhaps not unsubstantial understanding of the workings of society, would appear to know very little about himself. The social science enterprise has both form and mass yet, amoeba-like, this form is characterized by uncertain boundaries, while its mass has yet to be determined. In brief, any analytical or political focus on the social sciences is hindered by problems of identification and definition, and even more acutely by a paucity of data and a poverty of conceptualization in the area.

There is, however, evidence of a growing concern to subject the social science enterprise to a deeper degree of analysis than it has previously experienced – a concern that has been expressed by two distinct but interrelated movements. On the one hand social scientists themselves are beginning to examine the processes and institutions with which they are concerned, the growth of knowledge within them and its relation to the social and political environment – i.e. a move towards a sociology of social science (Crawford and Bidermann, 1969); while, on the other hand, a growing political pragmatism demands that social scientists should stand and be counted, that resources allocated to them be assessed, and that the benefits they provide, tangible or otherwise, be evaluated. It is from the latter direction, namely the political sector, that the demands for statistical data chiefly (or initially) arise. Statistics are seen to be required intranationally for the evaluation of ongoing programmes or for assessment of the *status quo*, and internationally to facilitate location in the league tables of national prestige – an area where frequently performance tends to be linked to position and figures tend to become disembodied from any appreciation of the significance of their source. There is indeed evidence that the influence of what Gross has termed the 'economic philistinism' of the statistical establishment, e.g. a preference for dwelling on the quantifiable and countable (Gross, 1966, p. 17), has penetrated the social science community to the extent that many efforts to assess the state of social science have been cast in statistics which refer to no concepts other than those that are numerically measurable. Hence attempts to obtain definition of the area and increase its visibility have resulted in adoption (and only infrequently adaptation) of statistical categories developed to assess the natural sciences. Some of the problems of assembling statistics for the social sciences were discussed at Paris by a round table meeting of conference participants and administrators. However, to place the discussion in perspective it is necessary to examine the earlier efforts in this area and to emphasize some of the difficulties that such efforts may explicitly or implicitly have involved.

PAST WORK ON SOCIAL SCIENCE STATISTICS

The three major attempts to assemble statistics on both the sources of support and the organization of the social sciences have been those of Ellis (1964), OECD (1966), and the Behavioral and Social Science Committee of the US National Academy of Sciences (BASS, 1969). Of these, only the OECD document covered more than one country, both the Ellis and BASS reports being devoted exclusively to the American situation. Since the BASS report to a large extent superseded Ellis's study and since OECD's effort stands alone as an attempt at crossnational assessment (although not comparison), it is best to restrict ourselves to the OECD and BASS documents and to relate them to their social contexts.

The OECD study was part of a larger attempt to examine and make recommendations on governmental policies for the social sciences. It constituted OECD's first venture into this area and, indeed, marked a departure from its previous primary concern with the natural sciences and their associated technologies in relation to economic development and growth. The 1966 report was however not OECD's first venture into statistical assessments of national scientific enterprise. Here, too, its approach had grown out of its concern with the natural sciences and from this concern resulted the publication of a manual entitled 'Proposed Standard Practice for Research and Development' (the 'Frascati' Manual) which was adopted by OECD member countries in 1963. The aim of this document was to measure research effort in terms of inputs of finance and manpower into research, the measurement of research output being excluded as too complex. The manual was therefore directed at facilitating internal and crossnational scientific assessments on the state of the natural sciences and was aimed specifically at policy-makers. The needs of the latter were seen by OECD as directed towards 'a few sound, clear defined figures that can be compared and contrasted to tell them something about science in their country, its resources and organization and on which they can base their plans for the future' (OECD, 1966, p. 81). Hence statistics for the natural sciences compare research expenditure and manpower across what was termed 'sectors of performance' (e.g. business enterprise, government, private non-profit, and higher education) by sector of finance, by scientific discipline, and by type of activity (e.g. basic research, applied research, and development).

The efforts of OECD in 1966 to apply the definitions and methods it had evolved for the natural sciences to the social sciences were not markedly successful. Data were lacking for many countries, while, further, what data there were could not be disaggregated from the categories in which they were originally presented into the categories in which OECD were interested. However, more serious than these technical difficulties, were certain conceptual and definitional problems, the most important of which were, first, the requirement to define what activities were covered by the term 'social science' and, second, the difficulty of uniquely categorizing what was or was not research. It was possible, the report concluded (when confessing its inability at that time to establish either meaningful or comparable statistics), that in the latter instance at least it might be better to consider a larger range of activities in the social sciences than to confine any analysis to a narrowly defined concept of research.

In contrast the work of the BASS committee was more modest in scope than the OECD survey, although when viewed in terms of finance and manpower, it was, within a single national context, a large-scale enterprise. The mandate of the BASS committee was to prepare a report on the present status and future needs of the component disciplines and joint research activities of the social sciences within the US. As part of this exercise, the committee attempted to assess the production and distribution of manpower within and across a variety of institutional bases and to estimate the total funds expended on social science research within a given period. This gave rise to two major problems. First, the difficulty of calculating resource expenditure on what could be termed 'development' (as compared with basic and applied research) in the social sciences and, second, the difficulty of evaluating the contributions of industry. Although figures were assembled for these two categories, it was admitted that considerable variation in these was possible and hence the total estimate could be regarded as being subject to significant error.

Reviewing the BASS findings in the *American Sociological Review*, Kenneth Lutterman (1970) noted that the primitive nature of the social organization of contemporary social science in the US was highlighted by the fact that the BASS survey constituted the first comprehensive attempt to assess the state of its development. It revealed that data on such basic questions as the financial support of research in a given discipline were not reliably available because of the current state of social organization of the social sciences; further, no detailed analysis had been provided of why patterns of support had developed or what the broad consequences of this had been. In addition, other unanswered questions included the need to assess the impact of these patterns on sociology and on the utilization of scientific knowledge, or whether in fact the source of funds made any difference (e.g. theoretical, methodological, or substantive) to the work performed. The need, stressed Lutterman, was for 'a basic sociological study of support and of the effects of funding on the development, theory, method and data for the behavioral and social sciences', and while perhaps one should not overemphasize fiscal concerns, it should be recognized that these formed a fundamental reality base for growth, development, and the national impact.

Lutterman's arguments highlight the dilemma alluded to earlier, namely the concern to link any statistical assessment with a theoretical understanding of the social sciences as a social product and to avoid the political demand for, and usage of, statistics to reinforce biases and to vindicate established positions (Bidermann, 1966). This dilemma may be seen to parallel, or indeed may be part of, the current problems within the social indicator movement. Here political pressures have created the danger of an overselling of the concept of indicators, and of ignoring the need to establish more modest objectives for statistical series based on firmer conceptual frameworks than are at present available (Sheldon and Freeman, 1970; Henriot, 1970). The thorny question facing the establishment of statistical series to evaluate the past, current, and possibly future state of the social sciences is therefore that of accommodating an acknowledged and significant political demand with the social scientists' need for conceptually based internal indicators (i.e. 'withindicators' of a system state in the manner of David Easton's 'withinputs'). In brief, one requires first and foremost to know 'what to measure and for what reason' (Bauer, 1966, p. 39).

In the discussions that follow a great deal of attention is paid to examining the operational difficulties of launching any national or crossnational system of assessment. Some of the issues raised (e.g. the problem of establishing a category for 'development') are familiar, others, namely the resource constraints in terms of time, money, and manpower needed to embark on efforts of this nature, or the requirement of political or institutional leverage to obtain information, are relatively new. However, most conference participants appeared to accept the need to assemble data along lines generated by administrative demands and hence it fell to Paul Lazarsfeld to question simply 'what is this data for?' The administrator's answer was presented by Jean-Jacques Salomon, who argues that the social scientist can serve both the policy-maker and himself by dredging out information at different depths and in different waters. However, this does not avoid factors such as the seductive nature of the quantitatively measurable (i.e. how can one account for factors such as quality in statistical series) or the problem of reification of statistical categories (i.e. to what extent should categories be treated as permanent fixtures). Pragmatically, such objections perhaps are of low priority; conceptually, with a view to establishing time-series to indicate the past and present state of the social sciences, they are undoubtedly of importance.

THE DISCUSSION

Introducing the topic to the Round Table, Elisabeth Crawford described the aims of organizations such as OECD or UNESCO to establish international and comparative statistics in the social sciences. The establishment of international standards is, however, only possible through collaborative efforts on a national basis, so in essence the impetus for collection and collation has to come from within each individual country. This presents the social scientists with the opportunity to act as pressure groups and exert their influence in establishing statistical categories which has in part been achieved by American social scientists with regard to the activities of the National Science Foundation, thus illustrating the chance for social scientists to occupy a significant role. Action of this kind is particularly important since social sciences are consumers of data whether it is used for research or policy. Hence, they can and should act as a pressure group on bodies, such as OECD, which are actively concerned with international standards and can exercise leverage on national data-collecting bodies.

OECD's growing interest in the social sciences was then outlined by Allison Young of the OECD R & D Statistics Division. Following earlier difficulties, more rigorous attempts are now being made to establish exactly what countries do in the way of assembling statistics for the social sciences and, perhaps more important, to ascertain exactly what activities they group under this label. From this exercise, it was hoped to be able to move towards the establishment of international standards. In reply to questions from other discussants, Miss Young agreed there are serious problems, particularly in using categories established for the natural sciences to cover the social sciences. It is possible that certain categories will have to be amended, but it was noticeable that countries that are at present collecting data on the social sciences are doing so principally on definitions framed for the natural sciences, with very few making either special provision for the social sciences or adopting special instructions to incorporate these new areas.

Expanding some of the points made by Allison Young, Jeremy Mitchell noted that after several years' experience in taking decisions in the UK Social Science Research Council, it was apparent that there are few sensible data on which to base such decisions. His view was that the kind of data needed should have three different dimensions:

first, they should be internationally comparable between different countries;
second, they should be comparable as between the social sciences and between the natural sciences and technology;

third, they should be collected on a continuous basis so one could get accurate measures of changes over time.

With these dimensions in mind, he had looked at the Frascati definitions (1963) as operated through OECD to see to what extent these could be adapted to the social sciences, in particular what kind of problems one faced on adapting these definitions, and to determine whether special categories were needed. The basic problems that resulted from this exercise were in part those noted before. The first and most obvious one is the distinction made in the natural sciences between basic research, applied research, and development. It is highly improbable that such a distinction would be satisfactory in the social sciences; hence, should we try to retain categories that were comparable with statistics already collected or should we devise special categories? There are also problems concerned with accounting for manpower, since in the social sciences it is impossible to use the same categories of scientists, technicians, and other scientific workers as in the natural sciences. Further, there are clearly severe definitional problems surrounding the social sciences, particularly in the industrial context – to what extent can pieces of 'research' be included that encompass social science methodology, survey techniques, or psychological testing but which many social scientists do not define as research? Market research is a good example of this and in the UK there is possibly as much spent in this area as in the whole of social science research. These then are some of the problems and possibly the only way to resolve them is to establish a continuing dialogue at an international level between social scientists and policy-makers. Such discussions took place prior to the drawing up of the Frascati Manual and possibly a similar arrangement should be encouraged to deal with the statistical problems posed by social science.

Further operational difficulties of assembling statistics were then discussed, especially those facing crossnational comparisons. Here, Eric Trist noted that when performing a survey of the social sciences for UNESCO (Trist, 1970), he had found that many Eastern European countries linked the social sciences and the humanities in the same statistical (and administrative) category. This makes any disaggregation of data extremely difficult. On this account, he was interested in a current convention being attempted by the UNESCO Science Policy Division where, in certain instances, rather than collecting aggregate statistics on the national level, they were attempting to collect data from key institutions in various countries. This measure is to be regarded as strictly a surrogate in any attempt at crossnational comparisons; however, it does illustrate that small-scale experiments must precede data-gathering problems on a macro-scale.

Responding to a question regarding the use of the 'development' category, Trist stated that in his experience this was relatively weak for the social sciences and he had not used it. However, attempts to measure 'development' are increasing, particularly in the US, where these are linked to measurement of effort on problems such as the 'urban crisis'. Agencies such as Health, Education, and Welfare (HEW) are currently attempting to build monitoring operations into their programmes; however, there are as yet no established norms of practice. Thus with the current emphasis on social policies, there is emerging an increasing realization that social programmes require evaluation and also possibly that engineering devices, such as pilot programmes, need to be introduced. These come near to constituting an analogue of development work in the social sciences and may also be linked with the emergence of a hazy but new concept through which social engineering becomes an accounting category.

Trist's approach drew queries from at least one conference member. Evaluation programmes for social development, it was stressed, required criteria of evaluation, and on this topic political sensitivities are high. As an example, in the Eastern Quebec project in Canada, great quantities of resources were invested in the enterprise itself but little on evaluation, this was primarily due to the political difficulties involved. To this Trist replied that he envisaged much of the work that he was suggesting being done 'in house', especially since the first steps entail the establishment of a collaborative relationship between social scientists and politicians. It is, however, worth while to attempt to focus some of the best minds in the social sciences on collaborative research in these areas.

Directing the focus of the discussion back to the problem of statistics and data collection, Orville Brim stated his concern for obtaining better information for the social sciences than were at present available. Essentially more refined data are needed and these are extremely difficult to obtain. For example, the BASS survey had cost half a million dollars, was heavily provided with manpower, and, since very little data on the state of the social sciences in the US had been available, the Commission had embarked on a detailed survey. They were able to do this since they had the power to obtain the required data from the various sectors. Yet, even though the data provided through the work were the best available, they were still inadequate. There was indeed, as Professor Trist and others had noted, an increased emphasis on programme evaluation within the federal government (e.g. 10 per cent riders for evaluation on all federal action programmes), and this and other efforts such as those of the Second Committee on Human Resources would result in more data, but even this was not satisfactory. Hence, future statistical efforts should proceed on at least two fronts:

(a) in terms of working reviews at an international level – to encourage and improve the data-gathering in the social sciences
(b) efforts on a national basis which might operate under somewhat lower constraints than might be true for more comprehensive studies. Such efforts might serve as models on topics such as manpower data or resource data for individual countries and could possibly be integrated at the level of an international body.

These suggestions led Jeremy Mitchell to stress the need to strike a balance between the data that people ideally would like to have and what continuous data one could actually collect, granted the gross insensitivity of the data-gathering systems in different countries. Unfortunately, systems are frequently clumsy and hence unable to work with the degree of refinement suggested. The more one refines one's categories in collecting data, the more one has to change them through time and this again destroys the value of the statistics. Hence some distinction should be made between categories involved in continuous procedures of data-gathering and the more refined categories developed for particular exercises with particular objectives, since in the latter case a much more sensitive system can be developed.

Dr Jenkins then emphasized the question of selecting carefully the appropriate level that various data-gathering exercises should take place on. Any agency or researcher must possess sufficient leverage on people or institutions to obtain the requisite information. Either one must operate from the level of the international body or from the national bodies themselves. The directives to people to produce information should come from these. Social scientists can undoubtedly contribute a great deal but chiefly at the level of concept development, as had taken place over the Frascati Manual. This would involve people discussing issues rigorously over a long period, but following this the final pressure for the implementation of their recommendations must inevitably come from a higher level.

Paul Lazarsfeld then intervened to applaud the Round Table's concern with the collection of data, but also to ask what are the data to be used for? There is a danger of information lying inert unless one sees that producing and applying it is an art in itself. This point should be drawn to the attention of governments. The fact that existing skills of applying social science data were underdeveloped could be illustrated from the experience of the medical field in the US. Here many government-financed health facilities are not supported by the poorer section of the community for whom they are intended. This is because modern health facilities constitute a bureaucratic structure that frightens the poor. Hence the problem is whether one should change the attitude of the man or the nature of the health facilities. Application is really a research problem in itself about which little is known. The mere collection of data leads to problems requiring more data and any recommendations for data-collection should at least indicate how one might link collected information with policies. This would also have to go hand in hand with the training of applied social scientists, people who (as had previously been stressed by Henri Mendras) should be equivalent to social medical doctors.

Much discussion turned on the question of whether statistics generated independently of any conceptual base serve any useful purpose. As Professor Goldschmidt put it, while general data are always of some use from the policy viewpoint, predetermined points of interest are required before detailed statistical work can be embarked on. Allison Young distinguished between the kinds of statistics that are to be collected on a regular basis and are expected to be internationally comparable and those that deal with special topics. The latter are not continually sampled but are examined once every five to ten years – pollution and health research are current examples of these.

Jean-Jacques Salomon, however, took up the problems of the collection and utilization of data in more detail. The first requisite, he thought, was to distinguish between two kinds of users of data. First, policy-makers at an international level who take decisions regarding the distribution of resources for specific purposes – these need statistics and need them badly. The morning's discussions illustrated the difficulties in obtaining statistics for the social sciences but even in the natural sciences the statistics were not very good and this was true not only on an international scale but often on a national level as well. However, decisions have to be taken and hence social scientists should exert a real pressure on national bodies in order that they should be involved in the process of decision-making and resource allocation. At present many countries are totally unable to evaluate their potential capacity, available resources, institutions, etc. The lack of a true evaluation of the present state of the social sciences in France is a good example here and probably the same holds for other countries as well.

The second aspect concerning the use of statistics is their use for social scientists, and this, M. Salomon considered, is another matter altogether. Indeed, these should be more sophisticated and more elaborate since they are required for the purpose of research *per se* – whether basic, or applied, or for the understanding of how the social sciences operate within a very broad framework. The quality of current statistics for research and development in the natural sciences are as good as can be obtained at present. Admittedly they are sometimes in error but even highly regarded economic statistics are far from perfect and many important economic decisions are taken on the basis of data that are open to challenge. Statistics that at present exist in the natural sciences should be considered a minimum and should not be misinterpreted. Such errors have in fact been made by some of the smaller countries with regard to the assumption, now known to be false, that a certain proportion of the GNP should be devoted to research and development. Also confusions sometimes arose; for example, between national and international organizations as to the correct collecting procedures for statistics. In addition co-operation is frequently difficult to achieve, particularly among international bodies. However, granted these difficulties, it is still essential to obtain common definitions and denominations. Perhaps one way to achieve this would indeed be a new Frascati meeting devoted to social science statistics, and if this was the case such a meeting should be convened as soon as possible before matters become very much worse.

References

BAUER, R. A. (ed.), *Social Indicators*. MIT Press, Cambridge, Mass., 1966.

BIDERMANN, A. D., Social Indicators and Goals. *Social Indicators*, Bauer, R. A. (ed.), MIT Press, Cambridge, Mass., 1966.

Behavioral and Social Science (BASS) Survey, *The Behavioral and Social Sciences: Outlooks and Needs*. Prentice-Hall, New York, 1969.

CRAWFORD, E., and BIDERMANN, A. D. (eds.), *Scientists and International Affairs: A Case for the Sociology of Social Science*. John Wiley, New York, 1969.

ELLIS, W. W., The Federal Government in Behavioral Science: Fields, Methods and Funds. American Enterprise Institute for Public Policy Research, Washington, D.C., May, 1964.

GROSS, B., *The State of the Nation: Social Systems Accounting*. Tavistock Publications, London, 1966.

HENRIOT, P. J., Political Questions about Social Indicators. *Western Political Quarterly* **23**, pp. 235–55, June 1970.

LUTTERMAN, K., Review Symposium on BASS Report. *American Sociological Review* **35**, pp. 338–41, 1970.

OECD, *The Social Sciences and the Policies of Government*. Paris, 1966.

SHELDON, E. B., and FREEMAN, H. E., Notes on Social Indicators: Promises and Potential. *Policy Sciences* **1**, pp. 97–111, 1970.

TRIST, E. L., Organisation and Financing of Research. *The Main Trends of Research in the Social and Human Sciences*. UNESCO, Mouton, Paris, 1970.

Part 3

Social Scientists and the Making of Social Science Policy

9 The federal government and social science policy in the United States

Henry W. Riecken

The important influence of cultural settings cannot be neglected in any detailed examination of the relationship between the social sciences and government. In this final section of the book, two chapters are concerned with the development of the social sciences in two sharply contrasting settings: the pluralistic atmosphere of the United States; and the People's Republic of Poland – an environment influenced both by long-term historical trends and by current ideological developments. Cultural considerations also dominate questions regarding the role that the social sciences can play within the new and emerging nations – a third chapter deals with this, examining some of the erroneous assumptions that, to date, appear to have dominated this area. Finally, the section is concluded with a short examination of the extent to which social science policy constitutes an area in itself – to what degree can a 'meta-policy' (i.e. a policy for making social science policy) be established?

In terms of sheer volume, both of resources and intellectual output, the United States dominates the current world picture of the social sciences. Has such a position been achieved through a deliberate policy directed towards the social sciences, or has it rather been an outcome of wider support for research and higher education within a constantly evolving institutional matrix? In this chapter, Henry Riecken argues towards the latter position. In a remarkably compact portrayal of the current state of the social sciences in the US and their wider linkages, he sees few criteria for the existence of a deliberate policy being met, other than those of the presence of men, organizations, and other resources.

Identifying the major actors and institutions concerned with the social sciences, Riecken discusses in turn the role of the universities, the operating agencies of the American government, and co-ordinating bodies such as the National Science Foundation in promoting the growth of disciplines and associated activities. He underlines the importance of examining the American situation from a pluralistic viewpoint and discusses the weaker power-base of the social sciences as contrasted to the natural sciences. Finally, three organizations seen as having special roles (the Social Science Research Council, National Research Council, and Russell Sage Foundation) are examined in detail with regard to their role in policy formation and in particular with regard to their influence in three recent reports concerning the present situation of US social sciences and the directions it might take in the future.

A social psychologist by training, Dr Henry Riecken is at present the President of the US Social Science Research Council. He was previously Vice-President of this body and before this Assistant Director of the National Science Foundation. He has taken an active part in much of the current debate concerning the organization and capacity of the social sciences in the US, and has written widely both on social psychology and on social science–government relations.

The notion of a policy – for social science or for any other purpose – implies a deliberate allocation of resources through means that are intended to achieve a chosen end. It also assumes the existence of resources – men, organizations, money, time, ideas – and suggests ways of using them effectively. Finally, it implies that there is agreement and collaboration among men and institutions to execute the steps of the policy.

By these criteria, the USA does not have a coherent social science policy. Except for one element – the existence of men, organizations, and other resources – the criteria for a *policy* are not met, although one can describe how resources are mustered and brought to bear on the activities of social science. Accordingly, this paper will be concerned with some of the ways in which US social scientists guide, abet, benefit from, and even reshape the actions and purposes of federal government agencies.

One further point of clarification is necessary. The US government does utilize social science in many ways. For example, the reports and recommendations of the Council of Economic Advisors, the analyses of the Bureau of the Census and the monthly reports on employment which flow from its Current Population Survey, and the Department of Labor's Manpower Report to the President all influence executive action and legislative proposals. The federal government uses social science to formulate and execute domestic economic policy. That does not, however, constitute a policy for the development of social science, which is the main concern of this paper. To focus on this aspect, primary attention will be given to social science in the private sector as it influences and is influenced by federal agencies.

NUMBER AND DISTRIBUTION OF SOCIAL SCIENTISTS

Let me begin by giving some idea of the size of the social science enterprise by pointing out how many and how diverse are the elements that would need to be co-ordinated if the United States were to attempt a social science policy. Another factor contributing to the difficulty of making a social science policy is the desire for autonomy felt particularly by the academic social scientists who make up the majority of the social science community.

There are about 110,000 active social scientists in the United States – if 'social science' is defined to include anthropology, economics, geography, history, political science, psychology, sociology, and statistics. About 60 per cent of them are engaged in university teaching, research, and service. Many of these are faculty members of the more than 150 universities that grant the PhD degree in one or more of these disciplines, or of the 600 or more colleges that grant disciplinary and professional degrees. Most are members of the 650 disciplinary departments into which these 150 universities are sub-organized (BASS, 1969).

It is not so clear where the remaining 40 per cent of American social scientists are situated. A substantial number are employed by federal, state and (more rarely) municipal governments as research workers, managers and administrators, and practitioners. It seems reasonable to estimate that governmental agencies employ about 10 per cent of the 110,000 while the remainder are distributed among industrial and commercial firms, non-profit research and service organizations, and various forms of private practice and consulting.

These manpower resources are very unevenly distributed among the various social science disciplines. By far the most numerous are psychologists and economists – about 30,000 of the former and 25,000 of the latter. There are perhaps 18,000 historians, 15,000 political scientists, and 12,000 sociologists. The other disciplines collectively number somewhat less than 10,000 members in the behavioural or social science component of the discipline. Looked at in terms of their employment, the disciplinary groups are also unevenly distributed. It is only psychologists and economists who turn up in sizable numbers in industrial and commercial firms, in private practice or consulting. Psychologists and economists are also extensively employed in government agencies, and political scientists and sociologists also occupy both research and administrative positions in government agencies. Nevertheless, the great bulk of social scientists are located within the academic community where a major share of their effort is given to education and training of future professionals. It is perhaps of incidental interest to note that these academic institutions produce currently about 4000 doctoral degrees a year and that this number is expected to rise to about 7500 by 1975. Within the academic community of social scientists, the occupational emphasis is heavily upon disciplinary education and basic research. About 70 per cent of academic social scientists in universities are primarily attached to one or another disciplinary department. Another 20 per cent find their homes in various professional schools, especially business and medicine. The remaining 10 per cent are mainly employed in a wide variety of specialized research institutes within the university structure (BASS, 1969).

FEDERAL AGENCIES SUPPORTING SOCIAL SCIENCE

This sprawling collection of autonomous units on the social science side is almost matched by the number and variety of federal agencies which encourage, support, or perform social science research and training in some form. The role played by these agencies is a major one, which increased very rapidly during the decade from 1958 to 1968 when federal funds available to the social sciences *increased* sevenfold from $40,000,000 to very nearly $300,000,000. The federal government contribution in 1968 represented just about 35 per cent of the approximately $803,000,000 expended for all research and development activities in the social sciences that year (BASS, 1969).

This federal support flows from a wide variety of agencies. Each of at least 25 distinct and separate agencies provided more than one million dollars a year for the support of social science research, either for its own sake or in connection with their particular governmental missions. A small number of agencies account for the preponderant amount of funding. There are four large ones that have had an especial impact upon social science research and whose budgets account for two-thirds of the total expended for research by the federal government in the latest fiscal year for which complete data are available. These four are the Department of Health, Education and Welfare – especially the National Institute of Mental Health and the US Office of Education – the Department of Defense, the Department of Agriculture, and the National Science Foundation (NSF). The contribution from the remaining nineteen or twenty agencies that support social sciences is not negligible however, and illustrates the principle, deeply embedded in the American political system, of pluralistic support. In the context of social science this means that many agencies support research that may take in a common disciplinary classification, for example, economics or sociology, despite differences in emphasis related to the missions of the various agencies. Thus, research on commodity markets supported by the Department of Agriculture and on wage structure by the Department of Labor are both properly called economics although concerned with quite different topics. Psychological research is also widely diffused among various agencies and, next to economics, is the social science most broadly supported by the federal government.

ATTEMPTS AT CO-ORDINATION

At first glance it appears that this vast array of performers and supporters results in a disorderly 'non-system', which would function only imperfectly, if at all. There is a measure of truth in this appearance. There is no effective single co-ordinating body, although various attempts have been made from time to time to construct one.

The National Science Foundation, which was originally charged with the support of science generally in the national interest, was also designated as the agency for the development of a co-ordinated science policy. The Foundation was not able to discharge this responsibility. The reasons are several. It was, in the first place, a competitor with existing agencies for power, for funds, for influence in the scientific community as well as in the administration. It was, in the beginning, far from *primus inter pares*. Starting with a very small budget and a tiny staff in 1952, the Foundation lacked the means by which to regulate or even influence its older and more powerful siblings in health, education, welfare, defence, and agriculture. Lacking immediate and direct access to the president, lacking legislative authority to direct, check, bend, or curb the scientific concerns of other agencies, short on financial resources with which to lure scientific talent, the Foundation was forced from the beginning to pursue a more indirect course, gradually building a case for the support of basic (as opposed to applied) research through scientific projects that were of lesser interest to the mission-oriented agencies though often of greater interest to the academic community. Taking as its charter the Vannevar Bush dictum that the basic research of today is the applied science and technology of the next decades, the National Science Foundation modelled itself after some of the more successful private foundations, making small grants in aid for time-limited projects in physics, chemistry, and biological sciences, almost entirely to scientists in academic institutions. Constrained by legislation from establishing any laboratories or research institutes of its own, and constrained by its budget from making block grants to universities or long-term commitments to particular investigators, the Foundation developed the project system to a considerable degree of perfection. Concern with the minutiae of individual research projects left rather little time for the development of overall policy guidance of science and, since that activity seemed foredoomed to failure anyway, little attention was paid to trying to co-ordinate the more influential and massive agencies in science.

Partly as a result of this and partly for other reasons, the specific responsibility for development of science policy was removed from the NSF in 1961 and granted to the newly established Office of Science and Technology (OST) in the Executive Office of the President. The OST was a necessary outgrowth of an office that had been established five years earlier – that of the President's Science Advisor. Initially the responsibility of one person, the demands of this position increased with the growth of the federal budget for scientific research and development until a substantial supporting staff was needed. The post of the President's Science Advisor (who is also the director of the Office of Science and Technology) has always been held by a physical scientist or engineer – Killian, Kistiakowsky, Wiesner, Hornig, DuBridge. They have been confronted by both massive and expensive problems of space exploration, military technology, pollution control, food supply, and by the needs of linear accelerators, large-scale astronomical observatories, oceanographic vessels, and holes to be bored towards the centre of the earth. These advisers, because of their professional background, as well as the pressure of other business, have not generally concerned themselves with the problems of the social sciences nor have they developed staff to fill that function.

Until very recently, there was no social scientist on the President's Science Advisory Committee (although that was recommended by an advisory group in 1962), and even now there is only a single social scientist member. The studies and reports with which the President's Science Advisory Committee concerned itself rarely included social scientists, even when the topics – for example, food or pesticides – touched very closely upon socioeconomic concerns. Thus, it is fair to say that for one reason or another the policy of the government in the social sciences has either been undirected or has been directed by physical and biological scientists almost inadvertently.

A third attempt at co-ordination should also be mentioned, though it was at least as unsuccessful as the first two in the social sciences, namely, the Federal Council on Science and Technology. This group, which consisted of representatives from within the executive branch (i.e. federal civil servants of below cabinet rank) was charged with responsibility for exchanging information and co-ordinating efforts among federal agencies. The Federal Council made one or two rather ineffectual attempts to review and assess the support of the social sciences but, by and large, it too confined itself to physical, biological, and technical engineering matters. Furthermore, like almost all representative groups of equals, it had great difficulty in making decisions that might affect the distribution of power and influence and it had, indeed, no overt and explicit mechanism of control.

Perhaps the most effective control mechanism is the bluntest, namely, the Bureau of the Budget, which is responsible for preparing the President's requests to the Congress for appropriations. This powerful instrumentality of the executive must adjudicate the conflicting claims of agencies, and sometimes of projects and purposes within agencies, for the always limited funds available. The staff of the Bureau of the Budget must, furthermore, act as the rather battered fender between the eager administrator of the federal agency and the President himself, interpreting the wishes of each to the other. This far from easy task is complicated by the fact that most of the Bureau staff are not professional scientists and must develop (the hard way) an expertness about funding of projects and tasks whose scientific merit is often difficult for them to assess. Although many of the Bureau's staff are themselves trained in one of the social sciences and have generally been sympathetic with the interests of these disciplines, they too are preoccupied with larger fish – space, military hardware, health, civil aviation, and so on. The development of a rational policy for the social sciences can claim only a small share of their attention.

Finally, Congress itself has had a role, albeit an indirect and unintentional one, in the shaping of social science 'policy'. For many years, a rather populist suspicion of social science and social planning (tending to confuse these terms with socialism) characterized the Congressional approach to a social science policy. At one point in the 1940s, for example, a sub-agency of the Department of Agriculture was specifically prohibited in its appropriation from conducting any further studies of rural community life – this because a particular study had raised some questions about the nature of social arrangements in one of the southern states. About the same time, there were also some questions raised about economic forecasting on the grounds that successful forecasting might have the effect of actually changing the 'natural market'. Such stultifying ideas seem largely to have disappeared from the present scene, although one can never be confident that some version of them will not re-emerge unpredictably during a congressional hearing.

When Congress was debating the language of the act that created the National Science Foundation, two rather distinct and strong views were taken. One was that the word 'science' was to encompass simply the 'hard' sciences, which have usually seemed to Americans to be more genuine than social science. That view would have excluded any entry of the Foundation into the social science field. The other view, which was espoused by scientists of all sorts and by some member of Congress, would have included the social sciences explicitly and specifically. Neither view prevailed in pure form. Instead, compromise language was adopted, which permitted the Foundation to proceed at its own pace in exploring and developing programmes in social science. This it did, commensurate with growth in its budget and development of some expertness on its staff, and with the very careful scrutiny of the appropriations committees of the Congress. The latter preserved for many years an attitude of suspicion and questioning towards projects in the social sciences and particularly towards anything that might be politically interesting or controversial. The Foundation found it prudent to defend its programme in terms of its basic nature, not claiming much societal relevance for the work of the scientists it aided. Such an attitude now has been swept away by the initiative of the committee (the Science and Astronautics Committee) with primary responsibility for the Congressional oversight of the Foundation. In 1965 this committee proposed legislation which the Congress enacted. It specifically included the social sciences and broadened the Foundation's authority in conducting applied as well as basic research. This very important step in the development of a social science policy is only being begun to be understood because of delays in implementing this enlarged authority, but it is clearly a significant move.

It was this same committee that took another step to generate policy advice for the conduct of its own affairs. It requested the National Academy of Sciences to create the Committee on Science and Public Policy, which could serve the Congress by providing an independent source of advice on science development.

The Committee on Science and Public Policy has operated so far primarily to commission reviews of scientific disciplines and topics. Characteristically, it began with physics and chemistry, and went on to astronomy, mathematics, and computation, but it did commission a study on the behavioural and social sciences which appeared in October 1969 (BASS, 1969). This study, which was sponsored jointly by the National Research Council and the Social Science Research Council, attempted to survey the present state, the accomplishments, the promise and likely developments, the needs and the means of satisfying them that the social sciences evidenced at present. Although the report of the committee that conducted this study was intended for the Congress, it is widely read and is expected to have an effect on the policies and programmes of the several executive agencies as well. The recommendations of the Behavioral and Social Sciences Survey will be considered below. They do not add up to a comprehensive policy, but taken together with other current developments they suggest a possible shape for one.

In summary then, the US presents the picture of a relatively large number of separate institutions both engaged in and supporting social science research without a single coherent co-ordinating body or a well-articulated set of regulatory institutions. At the same time that these enterprises are large relative to social science in the rest of the world, they are small, relative to the total body of science, in the United States. The efforts of social scientists have both benefited from inattention and suffered from suspicion that these disciplines were subversive of the *status quo* and might lead dangerously to new ideas. The development of a policy for these disciplines has been marked by a number of ineffectual attempts to co-ordinate them and by the proliferation of a 'non-system' of support and performance that is both ramified and complexly interconnected.

How well does this sprawling non-system work? What are the means by which it accomplishes whatever it does? What sorts of mechanisms urge it forward, impede it, link its parts?

PLURALISM AND FLEXIBILITY

It is not simple to characterize the nexus between social science and the federal government. One feature is obvious: the plural sources of both support and performance of social research implies the existence of many fibres linking the two sides. But the plurality of bidders and doers also allows for many alternative paths through the bundle of connections. Since there are many alternatives, there is some competition of ideas and purposes. A social scientist whose proposal for research on dyslexia is rejected as irrelevant by, say, the National Institute of Mental Health, can turn to the National Science Foundation, to the Social and Rehabilitation Service, to the Office of Education, or to the Institute of Child Health and Human Development. The agency that finds Professor X at the University of Z is not interested in research on methods of evaluating anti-poverty programmes can seek out another professor at a different university, or call one of the independent, private research organizations. Sometimes the agency can virtually create and wholly sustain a research enterprise, as the federal Office of Economic Opportunity did in the establishment of the Institute for Research on Poverty at the University of Wisconsin.

SYMBOLIC POWER DISTRIBUTION

Formally, of course, the power of programme decision and allocation of resources lies with the governmental administrative agency, subject to negotiations it must have with the Congress both as legislator and as appropriator of funds. But there is a third party involved, for, in most agencies, both programme and resource allocative decisions are made with advice from outside the government – most often on the part of committees composed of academic social scientists. Such committees are variable in the amount and kind of influence they exert, but it is fair to say that most of them have argued for the support of basic research and for the advancement of social science in its various disciplines. Thus, psychologists have been able to argue successfully for fundamental studies of learning under the aegis of mental health in much the same way that physicists have been able to justify the support of linear accelerators by funds appropriated for national defence. It is an interesting and instructive outcome of a social process whose intricacy was not fully appreciated (and whose outcome was miscalculated) by the scientific community at the time the National Science Foundation Act was being considered. Then there was substantial worry that federal bureaucrats would use the power of money to reshape the course of scientific investigation to suit administrative purposes. In fact, what seems to have happened to a large degree is the reshaping of administrative purposes to fit the course of scientific research. Some agencies, to be sure, have resisted this process and have actually persevered in supporting applied research and development directly relevant to a bureaucratically conceived agency purpose. On the whole, however, where the academic community has had a substantial voice, its wishes have been heeded, its needs met.

ALLIANCES OUTSIDE THE SOCIAL SCIENCES

Social scientists, whether within or outside universities, generally operate from a weaker power-base than do physical scientists and engineers, biologists and physicians. Social scientists have usually found it advantageous to form alliances with their more powerful colleagues, as the history of social science in the National Science Foundation and the National Institutes of Health well illustrates. There also have been coalitions with agricultural scientists and with engineers in the design of equipment and environments for space exploration, undersea research, and defence.

The liaisons, while certainly not conscious strategy on the part of the government or the academic community, can certainly be considered an example of the federal government's effect on the way the social sciences have developed. The scientific orientation of NSF encouraged from the beginning of its social science venture a positivistic brand of research. Quantitative, empirically oriented, experimental (where possible) research received the most favourable attention. Humanistic models of research, intuitive approaches, purely descriptive, historical accounts – as well as 'pure' theory, unrelated to empirically verifiable propositions – tended to take a secondary place. At the National Institutes of Health, somewhat the same attitudes prevailed, although much more consideration was given to 'clinical' research, after the medical model.

Neither agency encouraged research on politically controversial questions or other subjects that were, in the 1950s at least, considered to be none of the government's business – race and religion, for example. This reluctance was motivated by a sense that government agencies risked their impartiality in supporting such research and could scarcely avoid the appearance of taking one side in a controversy – in the eyes of the other side, at any rate. A certain political prudence *vis-à-vis* the Congress was admixed with this motive and, in the case of NSF, a rather strict interpretation of the fundamental charter of the Foundation to encourage only basic research.

The character of this alliance of social and natural scientists, and its effects on the growth of the disciplines, has been to emphasize a portion of these disciplines rather than to spread research and training funds evenly across the spectrum. Psychology, anthropology, sociology, and economics have received rather more attention than political science and history, for example. In recent years, the study of political behaviour has been assisted by federal agencies, and there has begun to be some attention to historical research that follows quantitative, proposition-testing lines. (More conventional history has had some help from a different federal agency, the Endowment for the Arts and Humanities, which has also announced its interest in those aspects of social science that are 'studied by humanistic methods'.)

Other kinds of alliances bred other problems: in agriculture, defence, and some parts of the Public Health Service, social scientists were drawn more narrowly than many would have liked into applied research whose objectives were defined by administrators or by applied scientists, physicians, and engineers. As a consequence, certain fields of research have been very heavily funded and well developed, e.g. human factors in equipment design, psychophysiology of vision, rural community sociology, agricultural marketing, ethnology of the Pacific islands and its western littoral – while such topics as industrial organization, urban communities, housing design, and the sensory apparatus of taste and smell have been virtually neglected, at least until very recently. As far as disciplinary emphasis is concerned, the applied, problem-centred nature of research in agriculture, defence, and public health has again favoured economics, psychology, anthropology, and sociology.

It is worth mentioning that numerous other federal government agencies employ or support social scientists *per se*: Labor and Commerce gives support especially in economics and statistics; Veterans' Administration in clinical psychology; the Office of Economic Opportunity, the anti-poverty agency, in sociology and economics; and a handful of small bureaux, commissions, and task forces in various fields. Social science in these agencies is mostly applied research.

Finally, it should be made clear that not all social scientists find the 'alliance' strategy congenial. Some believe that social sciences are not respected and will not flourish in institutions dominated by physical and biological scientists. Others think that the natural science model is a false one for social research, and still others seek an independent governmental organization for social science in order to achieve greater visibility and recognition. The social science community is divided on this issue. Another section takes the opposite view and believes that social science has benefited both intellectually and politically from close association with other sciences in government agencies. The debate between these points of view was well documented in the hearings on a senate bill to establish a National Social Science Foundation – an action which has not been taken, but remains a possibility (US Senate, 1967).

ORGANIZATIONS WITH SPECIAL ROLES

In addition to the universities, the operating agencies of government, and the co-ordinating bodies already mentioned, the social science scene in the United States includes three organizations that play rather special roles in regard to social science policy. Space permits only a brief characterization of each. All are private, non-profit-making organizations, which interact in diverse ways with the academic community and the federal agencies.

The Social Science Research Council was established in 1923 by a group of academic social scientists for the purpose of advancing the development of the disciplines. The Council operates through an extensive system of substantive committees, brought into being when and as there develops a consensus that some topic or problem needs and is ready to benefit from a concerted, often interdisciplinary, effort. The members of the Council committees are chosen for their special knowledge and usually come from a number of universities. The Council has, in its forty-five-year history, nurtured a wide variety of research and training tasks – from quite fundamental methodological questions to fairly applied ones. It is presently engaged, for example, in helping to develop better methods for the evaluation of compensatory education of disadvantaged children, and in assessing the state of training in foreign language and foreign area studies, both tasks being financed by the federal Office of Education. The Council also seeks private foundation funds to assist its committees in pursuit of basic research and educational tasks. For example, its Committee on Transnational Social Psychology will conduct a research conference on the conditions under which a dissenting minority in a group can be effective in changing group decisions and standards or norms of conduct. The Committee on the Biological Bases of Social Behavior is conducting short training programmes in biological research (both technique and substance) for social and developmental psychologists, sociologists, and anthropologists. Through such activities, the Council attempts to advance the 'state of the art' and to open up new directions in research. As already mentioned, it joined with the National Academy of Sciences–National Research Council to conduct the recently completed Behavioral and Social Sciences Survey, in part a venture into policy recommendation.

One of the many arms of the second organization, the National Research Council, is its Division of Behavioral Sciences, which came into being some seven years ago. This Council, which is chartered by the Congress and directed to provide advice on scientific questions to the federal government, is structurally somewhat similar to the SSRC in having a set of working committees composed primarily of university professors. Its tasks are somewhat different, however, and it is more directly linked to federal agencies through the advice-giving mechanism. Among the agencies to which it has or is presently providing counsel are: the Office of Education, for which it provides guidance and evaluates proposals for basic research on the educational process; the Bureau of Outdoor Recreation, for which it will plan and conduct a research programme on recreation and leisure; and the Bureau of the Census, which requires advice on research to illuminate some of the reasons for incomplete enumeration in censuses of population and to remedy these deficiencies. The Division also advises on the management and conduct of behavioural science research in the Department of Defense, through recommending strategies for improving both its quality and its relevance. The Division administers the Armed Forces NRC joint-committee on vision and a parallel Committee on Hearing, Bioacoustics, and Biomechanics. The Division of Behavioral Sciences also has a few activities which are not specifically advisory to any single US government agency, such as its Committee on International Relations in the Behavioral Sciences and its Committee on Demographic, Economic and Social Trends in the Western Pacific. The latter Committee serves the interests of scholars investigating problems of social, economic, and political development and modernization.

The third organization with a special role is the Russell Sage Foundation. It operates both as a grant-making and a research-conducting body, having a professional staff of a dozen or so who are actively conducting research, as well as a rotating group of three to five fellows who spend a sabbatical year in research, study, or in collaboration with the permanent staff. The Russell Sage Foundation has no direct or official connection with the federal government, but the talents of its officers and staff are drawn upon frequently to give the government advice in the social sciences. Its former president, Donald Young, was chairman of a National Research Council Advisory Committee on Government Programs in the Behavioral Sciences, which made a number of recommendations for the greater and more effective utilization of social science in and by the federal government (National Academy of Sciences, 1968). The current president of the foundation, Orville Brim, was chairman of a Special Commission on the Social Sciences established by the National Science Foundation, which recently completed a report on increasing the useful application of the social sciences in the solution of contemporary social problems (National Science Foundation, 1969). Other members of the Russell Sage staff have served in policy advisory positions concerned with the national census, the preparation of a social report and the development of social indicators, the prevention of crime and the improvement of rehabilitation. The Foundation has taken action in a number of areas related to public policy, for example, stimulating the introduction of social science into the education of lawyers and physicians; examining the social role of ability- and aptitude-testing in the American educational system; and the protection of personal privacy in social research.

These three interstitial organizations are important switching centres for the traffic between the federal government and the community of academic social scientists. To the extent that the US may be developing a policy for the social sciences, these organizations are helping to formulate it. Through their various study committees and advisory groups, as well as by the choices they make as to what fields or topics to emphasize, they have a place in the complex pattern of decisions that constitute the current strategies for developing and using social science.

TOWARDS A SOCIAL SCIENCE POLICY

It is significant that these three organizations have played major roles in the preparation of three recent reports on the social sciences, reports whose recommendations can be read as a sketch of what might be a national social science policy for the coming decade. These reports have already been mentioned, but it may be useful to examine the principal recommendations that they make, jointly and severally, for developing and using the social sciences. All three reports are, significantly, made to some portion of the federal government: the Behavioral and Social Sciences Survey (BASS), concerned with 'the present status and future needs of the component disciplines and their joint research activities', was directed to the Congress; the Special Commission on the Social Sciences (Brim Commission) was concerned with 'increasing the application of the social sciences in the solution of contemporary social problems' and directed to the Board of the National Science Foundation; while the Committee on Government Programs in the Behavioral Sciences (Young Committee) was aked to 'examine how the knowledge and method of the behavioral sciences can be brought to bear effectively on the programs and processes of the federal government'.

These three reports have similarities in purpose but differences in emphasis. They have consonant recommendations to make and, although no one report pretends to outline a comprehensive policy for social science, taken together they come fairly close to achieving one. By ignoring some variations in emphasis and by omitting some points made in only one of the three, it is possible to sketch the broad outlines of a social science policy on which there would be no substantial disagreement among the three recommending bodies:

1. There should be stronger representation of social science at the highest levels of science policy-making, that is the President's Science Advisory Committee and the Office of Science and Technology.
2. Government agencies should take steps to expand and improve the collection and dissemination, for research purposes, of statistical data about American society, and to make possible the collation of data from separate files at the level of greatest possible detail, while protecting individual privacy and anonymity of informants.
3. Social scientists should increase their efforts to develop a system of social indicators that covers a wide range of aspects of American life.
4. The National Science Foundation should give increased attention to and support for the development and utilization of the social sciences, including the improvement of education and training in the social sciences at all educational levels.
5. Social science research concerned with foreign areas (i.e. outside the US) should be supported by government agencies that have general scientific development purposes (in contrast to defence, commercial, or intelligence functions, for example), and wherever possible, such research should be conducted on an internationally collaborative basis, partly in order to further the development of the social sciences abroad as well as at home. A further purpose of collaboration would be to strengthen international programmes and organizations.

6. Measures to improve education and research in applied social science should include: (a) The establishment of schools of applied behavioural science, located at universities but not within or subordinate to disciplinary departments or professional schools; (b) the creation of social problem research institutes, with interdisciplinary professional staff, appropriate client-sponsors, and means for insuring a flow of qualified people through the institutes into the user agencies; and (c) the funding of a national institute for advanced research and public policy for the application of knowledge from all the sciences to the major issues of society.
7. The curricula of professional schools (law, medicine, business, social work, etc.) should include more social science instruction and knowledge appropriate to the profession, and greater emphasis upon social research.
8. Government agencies should support a broad spectrum of social science research, both basic and applied, both intramurally and extramurally, with respect to their own programmes and missions.
9. Federal government agencies should strengthen their staff competence in social science, identifying jobs for which social science competence is essential and granting leave to employees for advanced and continuing education.

Besides these nine points on which at least two of the reports agree, there are a number of more or less idiosyncratic matters which only one of the reports considered. It is somewhat more risky to assume that there would be agreement on their inclusion in a national policy for the social sciences, but in the absence of explicit evidence to the contrary they may be mentioned. The Young Committee recommend that the National Science Foundation give increased emphasis to institutional and departmental (in contrast to specific project) grants, while the BASS survey recommend long-term (more than five years at a time) guarantees of research support. The Brim Commission suggested that the effectiveness of community organizations should be evaluated and appraisal be made of opportunities to use social science in such organizations. The BASS survey suggested that social scientists undertake to prepare an annual social report on a private basis. The Brim Commission emphasized the role of social science, in adult education as well as in schools, and suggested greater opportunities for social science in business organizations and labour unions. The BASS survey recommended an annual increase of 12–18 per cent in federal funding for social science research and training.

Perhaps equally significant is that two of the reports (Brim Commission and BASS survey) urged that there *not* be established a Council of Social

Advisors (analogous to the Council of Economic Advisors) at this time, and one of the reports endorsed the establishment of a separate government foundation dedicated exclusively to the social sciences. The importance of these non-recommendations lies in the fact that legislative proposals for both matters lay before Congress at the time the reports were being prepared. The social scientists responsible evidently believed that there were other and better ways to use the social sciences in national planning and social development and they preferred to cast in their lot with other kinds of scientists rather than be singled out for special attention.

Overall, the tone of these reports is consistent – a heavy emphasis is on the desirability, need, and prospect of bringing social science into closer conjunction with the practical affairs of society. This is perhaps a response to the current awareness, widespread and uneasily accute, that all is far from well in American society, and the expectation that rational methods, grounded in scientific work, can help to steer the country through its troubles. Perhaps the emphasis on applied work comes from the desire to justify the expenditure of public monies on social science. Or perhaps it is the mark of an enterprise that feels its time has come. Whatever the source, it is clear that representative American social scientists are not so much dissatisfied with the practices of the past, which have been helpful in developing the disciplines, as they are eager and optimistic about their future prospects for a more important role in the affairs of the nation. They are proposing a social science policy that will help them to achieve this role.

Over the decades, but particularly since the end of the Second World War, the United States has evolved a pattern of strategies that has selectively, unequally, and without an overall plan, aided some of the social science disciplines to grow – even to prosper. Virtually at the height of governmental support for all science, social scientists were given an opportunity to outline what should be the influence of the federal government on social science policy, and they did so.

The extent to which the policies recommended by social scientists will be put into effect remains uncertain. It appears that the current atmosphere in government is less propitious than it was at the time these policy-recommending reports were being prepared. The social sciences are almost sure not to realize *all* of their ambitions in the near term in the United States, yet there are signs that great interest still centres on the possibility that social science may give some help to a troubled nation. For example, social scientists have recently been invited to work on problems of education, drug abuse, violence in television performances, law enforcement, and the administration of criminal justice – a range of tasks that will test their ability to make practical contributions to social policy and will surely have feedback effects on US policy for the development of the social sciences.

References

Behavioral and Social Sciences (BASS) Survey, *The Behavioral and Social Sciences: Outlook and Needs*. Prentice-Hall, New York, 1969.
National Academy of Sciences, *The Behavioral Sciences and the Federal Government*. Publication 1680, US Government Printing Office, Washington, 1968 (Young Committee).
National Science Foundation, *Knowledge into Action: Improving the Nation's Use of the Social Sciences*. NSB 69–3, US Government Printing Office, Washington, 1968 (Brim Commission).
US Senate Committee on Government Operations, *Hearings on the Bill to Establish a National Foundation for the Social Sciences*. US Government Office, Washington, D.C., 1967.

Interchapter

Henry Riecken's paper, which was read in his absence by Professor Rokkan, gave an extensive overview of the social science community in the United States and of those bodies with direct and substantial influence over policies affecting the development and organization of this community. This picture of pluralism, which so strongly characterizes the American scene, is contrasted sharply with the centralized policy-making that was later discussed by Professor Suchodolski from Poland.

This session and the two succeeding discussions on the papers by Friis and Dror examined salient aspects of the development of social science policy in different social and political contexts and of how social scientists themselves influence the development of policy for their own disciplines.

Following the introduction to Riecken's paper, Dr Brim, who had participated in the preparation of some of the reports that the author referred to, examined these documents as representations of the opinion of the social science 'establishment' on matters of policy that would greatly affect the development of their disciplines. Looked at in this light, the reports raise several interesting issues:

First, why did the social science community in the US argue against the establishment of a National Social Science Foundation and why did the commissions who had more time to consider the issue state that they were unprepared to recommend its establishment? This was one question that could possibly be examined against the experience of other countries.

Second, why did the commissions come out strongly against the establishment of a Council of Social Science Advisors when this appeared such an obvious point of entry into the White House for the non-economist?

And, finally, why were the graduate schools of applied behavioural science recommended in the BASS survey clearly opposed by the National Science Foundation?

Thus, although Dr Riecken called attention to points of convergence and agreement in the three separate reports, several of the issues on which the reports agreed raise general questions, while several on which they disagreed raise further questions as to what kinds of institutions were desirable. Replying to a query on the nature of co-operation and common policy between the social science disciplines in the States, Brim emphasized that interdisciplinary co-operation was excellent. There was virtually no competition between the disciplines and their objectives, and the agreement on broad outlines for development were almost unanimous. However, intradisciplinary harmony was possibly less marked, there being frequent problems within the disciplines themselves concerned not only with questions such as competition for grants and other scarce resources, such as prestige, but also with disputes over theoretical and methodological approaches.

Supporting Dr Brim, Eric Trist noted the remarkable change of outlook of social scientists in the US over the last twenty years. This change is reflected in the current reports, which, although presenting different angles of vision, all appear to point in the same direction. In particular, a large number of American social scientists are taking seriously the need to relate work in the social sciences to society. It will take some time before this re-evaluation, which in no way harms the development of the disciplines and the growth of fundamental knowledge, permeates the total social science system. However, the individuals and institutions supporting a re-evaluation of this nature constitute a valuable and influential body of opinion.

Einar Thorsrud, while welcoming Dr Riecken's description of the American situation, cautioned against applying its conclusions more generally and particularly to smaller countries. The author undoubtedly never intended that this should be done; however, we must not forget that in smaller countries with scant resources different research infrastructures are needed. Even in search of healthy pluralism it is foolish to allocate money to a large number of small institutes, and we can only move forward to creating desirable entities such as schools of applied behavioural science in such environments by co-operating (i.e. through institution building) on a multinational (e.g. Nordic) basis.

Orville Brim drew a sharp distinction between research institutes and organizations for training in applied social science. In the US, research institutes are well established, both linked with and independent of the university, examples of the latter being the Brookings Institution, the National Bureau of Economic Research, and the RAND Corporation. Proposals for schools of applied social science, however, raise considerable debate and do not meet with the easy acceptance that some members of the conference seemed to assume. Admittedly there have been moves from Buffalo and Syracuse Universities to establish separate degree-granting schools in applied social science, while other universities, such as Michigan, have attempted to transform their schools of public administration (an underdeveloped field in the US) into schools of applied social science. However, there is still substantial opposition among the social science community against such schools, chiefly on the grounds that their products will be inferior. Indeed, at present it looks as though almost everyone except social scientists wants schools of applied social science set up!

Differences of opinion amongst conference members regarding the need to build up schools of applied social science were brought out by Jeremy Mitchell. For him, the necessity for establishing such schools and institutes is not axiomatic. While in the UK in the past departmental rigidities have inhibited institutions of this kind from developing within university frameworks, we are now in danger of overcompensating for this. Unfortunately the idea of multidisciplinary work in the social sciences, particularly at the applied end of the spectrum, is rarely challenged; yet examples of really successful research in multidisciplinary projects are relatively few.

In response to Mr Mitchell, other participants saw the need within national structures for the establishment of an ecology of institutes ranging from fundamental to applied. Essentially different organizations are needed for different tasks, which implies a network of institutions located either within or independent from university structures. However, Henning Friis, after studying these problems for many years, has no clear-cut answers. In his own institution he does not force interdisciplinary teamwork; this comes sometimes from the inflow of personnel and sometimes from the nature of the problem. With such an approach people become gradually more and more aware of the other disciplines, a movement that is promoted further through staff seminars and similar devices. Can we train people specifically for this sort of enterprise? Professor Friis doubted it. We can provide an introduction, but much of the learning processes of applied research can only be obtained through experience. Nevertheless, the demands of such tasks are not (as had at times been suggested) at a lower level than those of a single discipline but are as severe as those of any research area.

Concluding the discussion, Professor Jolles wondered whether the clarity of Dr Riecken's paper disguised the complexity of the situation it set out to describe. Higher education is a centralized and highly political matter and this is a factor that frequently complicates discussions on suitable organizational arrangements for universities and research institutes. Hence, in contrast to higher educational establishments, the organization of research frequently had no tradition at all. Far from all countries being similar, each tended to have its own history and this diversity, together with the lack of a political dimension, must be carefully considered when discussing research structures.

10 The uses of social science in Poland

Policies for the social sciences

Bogdan Suchodolski

Information on the social sciences within Eastern Europe, on either their development or their current state, is remarkably limited. Linguistic barriers, scarcity of documentary material, and the low rate of mobility of scholars between East and West are all contributory factors to this situation, although currently such barriers are being significantly reduced (through exchanges of research workers, for example).

In this chapter, Professor Suchodolski fills some of the gaps by describing the historical antecedents and current orientation of the social sciences in Poland. His focus is on content and direction of activities, rather than on institutions and formal social science–government linkages, although he does trace the alliance between scholarship and politics through several centuries. In the pre-war period, social science in Poland was used as a tool in the struggles of various social groups, particularly in educational and social policy. Such factors are reflected in contemporary Polish attitudes towards the social sciences.

Suchodolski deals at length with the evolution of Polish social science in the post-war era, particularly Polish sociology, identifying the emergence of central problems as foci of attention. He examines the role of social science within a socialist state, drawing attention to some of the underlying assumptions that are made, and points to social science's growing importance within the educational system as a means of reshaping attitudes and actions. The role of social science, however, is limited and constrained by the influence and impact of other areas (e.g. the humanities) and hence the development of social science in any cultural context must be considered only as part of a larger system of educational and cultural activities.

Bogdan Suchodolski is a noted Polish theorist in the theory of education. He has written widely since the inter-war period on socialist education and its distinguishing features, and on topics such as philosophy of education and educational methods. He is attached to an Institute of the Polish Academy of Sciences in Warsaw.

THE TRADITIONAL SOCIAL ROLE OF SOCIAL SCIENCE IN POLAND

To grasp the present state of the social sciences in Poland, it is necessary to appreciate the vivid, if remote, traditions through which they have evolved. Throughout Polish history social knowledge has been an important factor in political action, even when it was still philosophical wisdom and keen observation, rather than science in the present day sense. The story has its beginnings in the Renaissance epoch.

The image of the Renaissance predominant in the history of social science thought has been reduced to the Machiavellian tradition of experience and advice, coupled with the Utopian tradition as represented by Thomas More at the beginning of the sixteenth century, and by Bacon and Campanella in the next one. Distinct from this image, however, is the great work by a Pole, Andrzej Frycz Modrzewski, entitled *De Republica Amendanda,* published twice in Basel by the famous J. Oporin in 1554 and 1559. The work was in Latin and it could thus evoke an international interest.

Modrzewski's position differed significantly from both types of thought then prevalent. He not only rejected the Machiavellian policy of force, trickery, and cunning as the inevitable product of ambition and greed for power, alleged to be inherent in human nature, but he was even less prone to take for granted the vague Utopian hopes which emphasized the prevailing state of social and political affairs yet was meaningless and unsatisfactory in offering advice. Instead, he wanted to present and vindicate a workable programme of restoration of the Polish commonwealth, and thus to set forth a model of an exemplary humanist state. He was confident that reason would lead the rulers to consent to rational political and social reforms, if enough reason was provided by an educational system with generally accessible schools, managed by competent teachers. His confidence is reflected in his own words: 'Let matters be settled', he wrote, having political quarrels in mind, 'by the court of reason, and not by that of impudence and perverse passion; let judges sit, who cherish the welfare of their country and the dignity of law more than profits, vengeance and godless power; who want law to exert its authority according to nature, and not for the sake of any party; whose intention it is to institute equal law for all living in this Commonwealth, instead of slavery for those of minor standing.'

Modrzewski was one of the first European writers who understood the importance of social knowledge – based on rational assumptions with underlying human values, and capable of critical analysis of actual relations – for practical, social, and political action. Fighting against the conservative camp in Poland, Modrzewski became for his own century, as well as for later ones, a symbol of the hope that theoretical vindication of the principles of justice might be an efficient weapon in the struggle for political and social reforms.

A similar historical experience was repeated in Poland in the eighteenth century. In its last decades there was a vigorous movement towards modernization of the feudal structure of the state. It succeeded, among other things, in establishing the first Ministry of Education in Europe, and in resolving the new constitution, known as the 3rd May Constitution. The essential meaning of the reforms thus introduced was to reconstruct the state ruled by the gentry into a state belonging to all its citizens. In the struggle for general education and democracy an important role was played by scholars and writers on social questions. Their inquiries into the social structure of the country, and their comparative disquisitions concerning other European countries, paved the way for partisans of reform and undermined conservative principles and obsolete notions. Furthermore, these men of learning often became politicans, party leaders, or high officials of the state.

The theories and activity of Stanislaw Staszic (1755–1826), in particular his concept of progress, reached well beyond the horizons seen by Condorcet, since Staszic related progress not merely to development of education and learning, but also to the successful struggle of the oppressed classes. The theories of Hugo Kollataj (1750–1812), with his 'physico-moral order' as a system of social ethics, deserve an equally high appreciation when compared with the Enlightenment moral philosophy. Both these men were conspicuous political personalities, who translated results of scholarly analysis into terms of practical reformist action.

Let us quote them. Staszic said: 'Knowledge inquires into the true relation of objects and men, and thus it digs an abyss under the system of violence and superstition'; Kollataj said: 'Human reason has reached two great ends: it has recognized fanaticism, and has been but little short of extirpating it completely: it has recognized despotism, and started to work busily upon its abasement.'

The Commission of National Education and the Constitution of 3rd May, the two great achievements of the alliance of scholarship and politics during the following century, were a symbol of the belief that progressive social thought constituted a forceful influence. Their example was used repeatedly in support of just social actions.

The third link in the chain of Polish experience with the use of social science took shape during the second half of the nineteenth century. Conditions were then peculiar. Poland did not exist as a state, but the nation's vigour in defying the alien powers was immense; governments were foreign, but it was the Poles who were still responsible for the fate of their nation. The main weapons they wielded in defence of national integrity were literature and art, seconded by history and social knowledge. Such knowledge had had many eminent representatives in Europe by then; Comte and Spencer had already laid the foundations of modern social sciences. Poland contributed to the general development, but sought its own methods, so as to serve the nation's consciousness and power of defence.

Thus social knowledge was directed towards the masses of peasants, the new industrial working class, and the intelligentsia emerging from among the gentry. Many sociologists co-operated with the growing peasants' movement that was channelling political and cultural advancement of the most numerous class of Polish society. Many others, like the eminent social scientist Ludwik Krzywicki, had been adherents of the emerging socialist movement; still others, like Edward Abramowski, became ideologists of syndicalism, which was soon understood, in the peculiar political conditions of the time, as a programme of national self-support. The conclusions of their differently oriented studies and researches were by no means uniform, but taken together they led towards a more or less consistent programme of social and educational endeavour for a modernization of the social structure of the country, for a development of democracy, and towards a modern nation.

Independence, won in 1918, opened up new opportunities for social science in Poland. Since that date there has been considerable development of Polish sociology. The name of Florian Znaniecki has been well known all over the world. Yet Znaniecki, for all his eminence, was by no means the sole personality in Polish social science of his time. He had many collaborators and disciplines, as well as many rivals and enemies. However, we are not discussing the various schools in Polish sociology, but their social significance, which was indeed far-reaching.

Sociological analyses served the paramount purpose of revealing the social structure and the sources of social conflict. Social research became a tool in the struggle for equal opportunities for various social groups, for political democracy, and for the levelling of economic privileges of the ruling classes. Research was focused upon disclosing the social ladder of the country. Other investigations dealt with fringe groups of those who could not find a job in Poland and were compelled into economic emigration, and with the unemployed whose number was sometimes large. Living conditions in industrial centres, in suburbs of cities in particular, were also investigated. In those studies various sources of discrimination and inequality were disclosed, the selective mechanism of the educational system, for example, with its difficult access to higher levels of education and professional careers. Special attention was paid to the situation and role of the rural population; to the obsolete agrarian structure and underlying class conflicts; to cultural aspirations of peasants and obstacles barring their realization.

Social research gave voice to public conscience, which was embodied in political vigilance. Further, it signalled imminent open or latent conflicts; appealed for a renewal of social and educational policies; or even backed the struggle of popular forces for the progress of democracy. The extent of influence exerted by social research differed in various fields, but was generally fairly considerable. It prompted a democratic growth of the educational system, and was instrumental in the making of progressive legislation and institutions in such fields as social security, medical care, and labour protection.

However, the role of social science in educational and social policy was not matched by its significance in other domains of public life. The vested political and industrial interests, as well as the state administration, were reluctant to acknowledge suggestions that might have been derived from social research. Scholars often withdrew to purely theoretical discussions which won some response among intellectuals, but which had hardly any practical effect on the larger population.

This brief historical sketch seems to be a relevant and necessary introduction to modern problems, which will be our main concern here, as it allows for a better understanding of important factors underlying the contemporary Polish attitude towards social sciences. Indeed, no nation can form its image of social sciences out of a historical void, and its policy towards them must reflect those values and expectations that have been taken for granted and held in esteem in national awareness during its historical development.

THE NEW SITUATION AND NEW TASKS IN CONTEMPORARY POLAND

After the Second World War Poland set out on its way towards socialism. Agrarian reform was proclaimed, landlords' estates were given over to peasants, and, sometimes, state farms were established; industry and commerce were nationalized, with a narrow margin left for private enterprise in small trade and the crafts; political power and administration were largely committed to the population led by political parties, among which the major role has been played by the workers' party; education was made virtually accessible to all; new prospects were opened up for further economic and cultural development of the country, accelerated by social reforms which mobilized the latent forces of the nation.

The new situation established fresh tasks for social science. The assumption underlying the socialist programme is that natural forces as well as social processes will be increasingly mastered by humanity, which means that conscious handling of life-conditions will be increasingly rational and efficient. The programme of socialist reconstruction was to be brought into effect within new political borders, with several millions of inhabitants of the former eastern provinces migrating to the recovered western territories. Another factor arising from large-scale migration was the onset of the process of accelerated industrialization, moving people from rural areas to urban centres. At the same time, the lack of class barriers to higher levels of education resulted in the gradual disappearance of the former divisions between the enlightened strata and the rural and urban working classes, as well as between manual and white-collar occupations. The new political and administrative structure gave more political and managerial power and responsibility, and demanded more sense of public involvement, from more people.

This changing social reality was becoming an increasingly interesting domain for social research, while practical postulates entailed by the socialist ideal constituted a challenge for sociologists to make their knowledge more useful in the practical moulding of social and economic policies.

Social research covers an increasing range of theoretically significant and practically important problems. Some of the research topics are: migration processes; the disappearing of old and emerging of new social links; social effects of rapid industrialization, such as the emergence of completely new industrial centres; psychosocial processes in industrial workers newly arrived from rural areas; maturation of the young generation and its involvement in adult life; changes in family life and structure, and of neighbourhood links, in large cities; the mass cultural processes such as the influence of radio and TV; and (descriptive) studies of various occupations and professions.

Within such an extensive range of investigations some central problems are slowly crystallizing, attracting an increasing number of scholars and integrating numerous and varied efforts. These central problems emerge from a variety of empirical investigations made in different university centres as a consolidated effort with common themes. Among them are industrialization and urbanization processes; organization of and attitudes to work; mass cultural phenomena; restructuring of rural economies; and social relations in rural communities.

At the same time such concentration of effort led from small-scale research on objects such as a single township or enterprise to surveys of larger processes of social change. Such shifts from micro-analysis to a synthetic approach has recently been typical of Polish sociology. The most general and controversial aspects of social structure are investigated, such as changes in the class and stratification system, problems of the shaping of a socialist industrial society, the growth of democratic organizations and institutions, and mass cultural processes as distinct from those typical for capitalist countries.

Underlying all these efforts is the most general question: taking for granted that socialist and capitalist types of civilization employ similar technological, scientific, and even organizational means, and that their growth is in many ways similar, and involves such processes as industrialization, urbanization, development of democratic structures, and the emergence of mass culture – to what extent and in what ways does socialism bring about new social and human values?

THE ROLE OF THE SOCIAL SCIENCES IN MOULDING SOCIAL AWARENESS

There can be many social uses and influences of results of social research. Without attempting any detailed classification, it is possible to point to the role of research in the shaping of social awareness as different from its significance as a factor influencing actual action.

The shaping of social awareness has been an important task ever since the war ended. Generally speaking, it has been necessary to try to eradicate those attitudes and notions that have their roots in the social reality that is no more, while it has been no less urgent to promote concepts relevant to new forms of social relations. It is well known that in post-revolutionary periods social consciousness more or less lags behind social reality suddenly reshaped by arbitrary legislation. It has been necessary to inform, persuade, and educate people to see reality as it actually is, to understand the principles underlying new institutions, and to grasp the new ways in which political mechanisms function.

In this extensive educational effort, the major burden of which has been laid upon the school system and the mass media, social science has an important share. Its task is to gather data about, and to formulate diagnoses of, the new aspects of social relationships. One type of sociological initiative has been the promoting of dozens of competitions for diaries and memoirs about the recent quarter century. Materials thus obtained have been subject to analytical studies, but much of it has been published and has become favourite reading for large groups of individuals who recognized their own experiences in the memoirs of others.

This type of material shows various aspects of social life with a subjective bias of personal feelings, ambitions, successes, and failures. Its counterparts have been empirical studies – with an apparatus of statistical analysis making up for the subjective element inherent in such tools as questionnaires and interviews. Such studies deal most often with conditions of life, human interrelations, and the functioning of various public institutions.

Thus, there have been two ways of arriving at an adequate image of the new social reality: individual reports, concrete and vivid but subjectively biased; and more abstract but objective schemes and models attained by systematic research. The social sciences as a source of information and diagnosis have been accompanied on one hand by serious journalism and by realistically minded literature; on the other, they have been seeking theoretical generalizations and a prospective interdisciplinary synthesis of the new social reality.

The second function of social science may be called an apologetic and unmasking one, with reference to practical conclusions that must be drawn from research results. Apology appears to be incompatible with an exposing of faults. However, it is peculiar to the role of social science in Poland that it could sustain the difficult balance between the two. Social research in this country has been 'apologetic' in that it takes for granted socialism as a form of social life intrinsically more valuable than the capitalist one; however, at the same time it can be described as blame-seeking or critically oriented, because another underlying assumption is that socialism is evolving and thus subject to improvement in each moment of time, and in each of its institutional aspects.

Obviously, both functions remain in a state of mutual opposition and tension, but this is desirable in order to prevent the apologetic tendency from degenerating into non-scientific dogmatism, and to keep the critical tendency from passing beyond the justified limits and into barren destructions. In general Polish sociology has avoided both these dangers on its difficult but important and useful course. By instilling knowledge and imparting attitudes it has helped to educate people for modern tasks and for more extensive participation in public life and leadership.

This type of activity has been conducive to the fulfilment of sociology's third task – that of moulding the social thinking and imagination of the community. Social research, besides presenting a dynamic model of reality, is supposed to help people in a reshaping of their thinking, attitudes, and actions.

This is an important issue. We have to realize that the ways of thinking and reasoning of the larger educated public, as distinguished from that of professional scholars and scientists, is a social phenomenon shaped under the preponderant influence of the fact that in various epochs various scholarly disciplines have acquired a dominant significance. In the nineteenth century it was mathematics and the natural sciences that formed the image of education. The second half of our century is a period marked by a growth of the social sciences, while social issues are becoming all important throughout the world. Hence, it seems justified to believe that stress ought now to be laid on social thinking as the new important element in liberal education.

Social science in Poland has assumed such a responsibility. It constitutes an element of school programmes on various levels; a share of social knowledge is administered in elementary schools, and is obligatory to all children; in high schools, as well as at university level, there are lectures and classes initiating the young into theoretical and practical aspects of contemporary social knowledge and social life.

Promulgation by mass media is another outlet for social knowledge. It has coverage in the daily and weekly press, in radio and TV programmes, and in series of lectures organized by various institutions for popularization of social science and adult education. Sociological ways of thinking are thus becoming more widely and thoroughly familiar. Of course, only a few are interested in the technical theories or conceptual structures of professional sociology, but there is a large and increasing group of political, cultural, and labour administrators who need and look for a more simple and condensed version of social science.

In this connection the fourth task for social science becomes evident. There is a general interest in the future, recently acknowledged in an interdisciplinary effort to draw up an image of what the country will be like by the year 2000. Social scientists have a major share in this endeavour.

They promise to establish certain trends in development, and to point out the ways to consciously and purposefully shape them. Involved here are such processes as changes in the social structure, modification of local environments, evolution of new forms of work and organization, emergence and disappearance of various aspirations, attitudes, and types of cultural participation.

This type of investigation and forecast appears as a new and significant element of social consciousness in a nation sensitive to the dynamism of growth. Social science provides intellectual tools and working suggestions in an effort to visualize and meet the challenge of the future.

PRACTICAL IMPACT OF THE SOCIAL SCIENCES

In addition to their role in influencing social awareness, the social sciences are directly useful in organizing group action. Modern society is a complex whole of diverse but interrelated elements; it provides an institutional framework for human activity whose efficiency depends upon the level of organizational structure and its ability to make proper use of individual motives and involvements. The social sciences contribute to more efficient functioning of such a structure by uncovering its latent mechanisms. The achievements of Polish sociology in this field are remarkable and highly appreciated by those who make practical use of them.

In the first place, one can think of the investigations into work organization and the situation of industrial workers and employers. Processes of industrialization are still relatively new in Poland, and they are still increasing. Sociologists have been keen to turn their attention in this direction. Industrial sociology has covered a wide range of problems of vital importance for industrial managers and executives, as well as for workers.

Social research helps to improve management systems, particularly those elements that involve the human relations aspects of decisions, which are sometimes critical for the efficiency or failure of managerial endeavours.

At the same time, social knowledge is an essential element in programmes of executive training at all levels. In a modern company technological staff, besides handling technological processes, must handle people as well, and thus some psychological and sociological training is vital for an engineer, who is expected to be capable of promoting an atmosphere favourable for team-work and for the sustenance of positive attitudes to work.

The third field for industrial sociology concerns problems of wages policy and of economic incentives, and issues of social policy such as work and leisure conditions; protection of health; old-age security system; as well as human problems of recruitment, advancement, and rewarding of workers.

Results of sociological investigations are transmitted to industrial organizations by the publications and special reports of experts. But though these two ways are used and appreciated, big companies have recently started the practice of employing their own sociologists on full-time research and in counselling posts. The character of their work varies depending upon their own personal bent, and upon their relationships with managements and workers; co-operation is sometimes far from harmonious, but in other cases it is fruitful. The role of an industrial sociologist may be that of an expert, or he may act as an officer for special tasks, or he may assume patterns of activity modelled on labour leaders. All these are important and novel forms of transforming social knowledge into practical action.

There are other fields where social research is equally important, though in a less conspicuous manner. For example, urban and rural sociology; environmental planning; sociology of leisure; and sociological problems of education and health. Many of these various efforts have been recently integrated within surveys of industrialized regions.

Processes of industrialization in various regions involve many complex problems of spatial planning of factories, living and recreation areas, communication networks, migratory trends, education, health, and cultural services. A sociologist's voice in these and other matters, however important, by no means carries equal weight to that of the industrialist. Sometimes growth is spontaneous and arbitrarily legislated by an administration working without any far-reaching design, but in other cases plans are elaborated by teams of experts, including sociologists.

However, the role of sociologists in these domains is not yet clearly defined; something more is required than casual counsel or an expert opinion in an emergency. As it is, sociologists cannot feel responsible for whole enterprises, while managers are not qute convinced that they should give an ear to sociologists' suggestions. Tighter forms of co-operation, and more systematic use of social knowledge, would be advantageous for both parties.

However, the practical importance of social science is by no means exhausted by the help it gives in improvement of local organizations, institutions, and endeavours. Underlying all these situations are more general principles and assumptions, and in each individual case nation-wide decisions are reflected in a variety of ways. Micro-sociology must always point to full-scale or macro-sociology. Sociological investigations in Poland are directed so as to lead through empirical analyses and case studies to general concepts, allowing for the formulation of universally valid principles of economic, social, educational, or cultural policy.

Thus, for example, studies on industrialization serve not only practical purposes, but they also cumulate in general conclusions about the nature of socialist industrial society. They show how the functioning of a social system of industry shapes communities, institutions, social stratification and class divisions outside of industry. Similarly, studies on work and management systems lead to more general conclusions about the larger social system in which work and power are distributed in certain ways. The same can be said about several studies on state and regional administration, labour and regional self-government, participation of citizens in power and control.

However important the voice of sociologists is in all these matters, there are other factors that are decisive in decision-making processes and the exertion of power, e.g. responsibility for the structure and nature of authority are political factors. Even though Polish sociology, particularly recently, has been taking into consideration problems of state and of politics, still its role here is limited to a description of the actual reality and to exposing its trends of development. It does not intend to give advice or suggestions, and indeed it could hardly be expected to do otherwise. There has never been any example of a state governed by sociologists and it might be doubted if such a vision for the future would be a tempting one.

ALLIES AND OBSTACLES

Discussion of the role the social sciences play in shaping social awareness has repeatedly exposed certain limitations for this role. The social sciences are an important, but by no means the unique, source of knowledge about man and society. At this point it is not possible to enter into the interesting discussion of the scope of the notion of the 'social sciences', and their particular relationships with other disciplines dealing with man and his forms of social life. These issues have been differently settled in various countries. It should be stressed, however, that any analysis of the role of social sciences in collective awareness cannot avoid questions about a similar role played by disciplines such as history, philosophy, ethics, psychology, and pedagogy. The relations of the social sciences with these disciplines are closer in Poland than in a number of other countries and this is reflected in the accepted usage of the term 'social sciences', which covers all the humanities, as distinct from the English usage for example. As will be pointed out, such terminology also underlies the organization of science in Poland.

It therefore appears that various disciplines collaborate in shaping collective awareness, and that any definition of the functions of the social sciences ought to account for this fact. Analysing their role from this standpoint, it may be concluded that their relevance pertains mainly to intellectual contents of collective awareness. The social sciences reveal the reality and explain its structure and its trends of development; their role in motivating behaviour, and in forming prospective images and intentions influencing the choice of values, has been minor in comparison with other humanities, such as philosophy, history, etc. It is the latter that influence attitudes, inclinations, and aspirations in a direct manner.

However, little is known still about human nature and personality-forming factors, or about mass changes in appreciation of the forms and objectives of life. People, in our country, are apt to believe that social sciences are only partly responsible for the processes of mass attitude formation; general education and massive cultural participation seem more crucial for the evolution of a certain new set of vital values.

At this point one arrives at the limits of feasible and efficient intervention of science into the collective and individual lives of people; beyond it extend the regions of creativity and spontaneity, unpredictable and invulnerable to scientific control. It is in those regions that new values and attitudes are born, which can be subject to purposeful manipulation only after they become social facts. People are capable of cultivating biological life, even though they cannot produce it; similarly, they are capable of guiding the social and cultural development, even though its creative elements defy any planned control. It was not socialism that organized the masses by any scientific elements contained within it; rather it was the revolutionary labour movement that gave birth to the socialist theory as its weapon. Having this in mind, Marx wrote, 'philosophy finds its material weapon in the proletariat, and the proletariat finds its spiritual weapon in philosophy'; and he added, 'philosophy is the head, but the proletariat is the heart'.

To avoid exaggeration in our judgement, these words should be remembered when discussing the role of social sciences in moulding collective awareness. While appreciating their significance in introducing important knowledge into social thinking, one ought to remember numerous other factors that shape other regions of social consciousness, or the 'heart' of the people, their values and aspirations as an expression of a definite ideal of life.

This is clearly understood in Poland. Together with a growing awareness of the educational role of the social sciences, there is a discernment of the function of the larger system of educational and cultural activities, and among these the human disciplines mentioned above, as well as of reality itself, as stimulating and reshaping motivations and patterns of social behaviour.

Limitations of the role of the social sciences for practical action can be shown in similar terms. Practical sociology has many allies and as many obstacles to overcome. Social reality is obviously shaped to a considerable extent by the legal and economic disciplines. The sociologist's role is in most cases reduced to that of an analyst and a medicine man. Lawyers and economists, rather than sociologists, are those who are in a position to exert effective influence, though sometimes the latter are also invited to co-operate.

The links between sociology and law are particularly well established and promising. Recently, too, serious efforts have been made to establish closer relations between the social and economic disciplines. It is believed that a one-sided economic viewpoint cannot be sufficient for the formulation of the socialist programme of development. Economic policy must take into consideration not only its own narrow logic, but also the social processes on which it depends and which in their turn depend on it. Directives for action must be defined by joint efforts of economists and social scientists. This is by no means always a matter of course; sometimes open conflict emerges between purely economic directives based on profit considerations and sociologists' schemes to promote social welfare.

However, as has been the case with respect to shaping social awareness, and also in the field of practical influence, not only other scientific disciplines compete with social sciences, but also forces directly shaping social life. We mean here political forces in general. Politicians who wield power, and those who are responsible for the general principles behind the activity of the state, make the decisions in matters of long-term goals and strategies. Economic and social, educational and cultural policies are decided in power centres; in those centres decisions are taken as to the distribution of national income, and as to proportions allocated to individual and collective consumption. The daily life-conditions of the people, their opportunities, and their expectations are thus formed for them.

The social sciences operate within a reality that is already moulded. Could it or should it be otherwise? An affirmative answer is by no means obvious. Some sociologists do feel a yearning or desire to direct the most essential aspects of social life, i.e. to establish its objectives and its strategies, but the bulk of them adhere to a more humble concept of the tasks of social science, or for their limitation to the sphere of technical solutions. A sociologist becomes increasingly attracted to the role of expert, ready to suggest how to do best what must be done, but reluctant to answer the question, what ought to be done. Though there are people who are opposed to a reduction of social knowledge to sociotechnics and though researches are developed that have no technical import, still the narrower image of a practical role for sociology seems to overwhelm the more traditional notion of sociology as a social philosophy pointing to remote ends and values of the collective human life.

POLICIES FOR THE SOCIAL SCIENCES

The development and growing influence of the social sciences in Poland have long given rise to many organizational and financial problems. What resources ought to be assigned to them? What sort of research ought to gain priority? How should the principles of collaboration of the various branches and centres of the social sciences be established? What relations should there be between theory and practice, how ought research results to be transmitted and put into action?

To some of these questions answers can be found in the general system of financing science in Poland. This is done by the state through higher education institutions and the Polish Academy of Sciences. The social sciences receive a share from both. Other sources are of minor significance, though recently large industrial enterprises and local authorities have been ready to pay for some sociological research.

However, the financial problem is not an acute one for social sciences in Poland. Their resources are mostly sufficient for research and training, and for publications. Editorial output in social science is relatively large. Like any other developing discipline, sociology would welcome an augmentation of its means, but lack of money is not a serious limiting factor.

A more important limitation is a strategy for development. As has been mentioned, the social sciences find their place within the Polish Academy of Sciences in a section of this name (the Social Sciences Section) together with all the humanities and historical disciplines. The name of the section reflects a conviction that a social standpoint ought to prevail in historical investigations, in linguistics, and in the science of literature, in pedagogy and psychology, in legal and economic disciplines. Such an attitude is meaningful both theoretically or methodologically, and from the practical standpoint of defining their roles and tasks. That their way of thinking dominates is a token of a victory for sociologists.

However, it is of vital importance to be interconnected with other disciplines. Various and sometimes promising efforts are made in this direction. Yet, this is a painstaking job. It is easiest in the well-defined practical branches of research, such as industrial and work sociology, sociology of science, sociology of education, but much more difficult when theoretical considerations on the whole of social life are involved, as is claimed by various disciplines.

Recently new perspectives have been opened up because of the establishment by the Academy of Sciences of a special committee for elaborating on development prognoses for the country. In the committee named 'Poland 2000' various experts are grouped – demographers, economists, geographers, educationalists, and, of course, sociologists. The latter are expected to work on the following problems: social macro-structure (social stratification and class structure, changes of social structure in urban and rural areas); social micro-structure (with emphasis put upon family, local communities, residential areas, social pathology); problems of work and industry (effects of automation and of technological progress, structure of labour and management); socialist institutions (national councils, self-government, planning, administration); value and aspiration systems and the impact on them of scientific and technological revolution; and cultural changes.

This programme of research, integrated with economic investigations on income and consumption patterns, with geographical surveys on spatial planning, with pedagogical and psychological studies of modern education, defines the main line of research for the social sciences seen as particularly important by the state authorities and by other sciences.

It can be hoped that in the future substantial manpower and resources will be allocated for this programme. This does not mean that other types of research will be abandoned; in the Institute of Philosophy and Sociology of the Academy, as well as in university sociological institutes, the full scope of investigations characteristic of modern social science in Poland is directed towards the effort of visualizing the future of the country.

We believe that not only will such vision be important for social and economic planning for the coming decades, but, in addition, it will entail a rich theoretical perspective concerning assumptions and criteria underlying long-term predictions. We also believe that the prognoses will bring solutions to the most difficult problems concerning the nature and character of the future socialist society, in which industrialization, urbanization, and democratization processes will take on a new shape.

Interchapter

In introducing his paper, Professor Suchodolski stressed four interrelated questions. What is the role of history in the development of a nation; what are the role and importance of contemporary social problems; what role can social science play in the reorganization of contemporary social life; and what are the limitations of the social role of the social sciences? Are the social sciences the major means available to shape society's future or would it be preferable to leave this in the hands of the natural sciences and technology?

The discussion arising from this paper takes up two significant issues, namely the question of centralization or decentralization of control for social science research and teaching, and on a wider level cultural differences in the development of the social sciences within different national contexts.

The topic of centralization was first broached by Andrew Shonfield, who wondered what degree of centralization is appropriate in the management of different areas of the social sciences. Professor Suchodolski's account of the special features of Poland supports Shonfield's knowledge of other countries of Eastern Europe where economics is hived off and treated as more scientific than the other social sciences. Is this part of the great Marxist tradition of singling out economics as a clear guide to the rules that direct social development? The effect of the different types of organization in East and West is that in the East a certain type of decentralization has occurred almost by accident (because of the feelings held on the ideological role of the social sciences), while in the US decentralization is due to other factors. In Britain the Social Science Research Council exists to channel public funds into the social sciences, treating all the disciplines together. However, this does not obviate difficulties in central management, particularly the funding of interdisciplinary studies. The almost instinctive recoil from central pressure to introduce interdisciplinary work may reflect genuine epistemological differences among the disciplines. So far we have not found the answer to this.

Professor Suchodolski was asked whether Poland has central coordination of work in the social sciences and central provision of funds, since this appears to be an important point of policy. Thus, while it is principally a pragmatic decision whether work is commissioned in one or several spots, it would be informative to know how much *central* decision-making there is, especially in comparison with the US, where there is little, if any.

Professor Suchodolski replied that in Poland, as in France, there was a strong tradition of centralization. At present there are marked attempts, especially within the universities, to achieve cultural and scientific decentralization. There are also attempts to decentralize the Academy of Science; although these are causing severe problems. Hence, while the intellectual possibilities are there, efforts to decentralize face difficulties. The university system also poses significant problems, inhibiting efforts directed towards common programmes of research. Professors can meet to arrange collaborative efforts, but seldom do so. The cause of this was the federated structure of Polish universities which provided many professorial chairs all of which act as separate centres of decision. Each professor is, by tradition, autonomous and in charge of his discipline, hence it is difficult even to arrange any system of cross-departmental credits for students.

Professor Kredar then asked what reasons might motivate moves to either centralization or decentralization. An illustration existed here in the recent history of the social sciences within the US National Academy of Sciences (NAS). Under the presidency of Detlev Bronk in the early 1960s, the NAS had attempted to unify and centralize the social sciences within its structure. Previously only one or two of the social sciences were formally represented in the Academy (e.g. anthropology and psychology) and it was decided to bring in the other disciplines. This effort at first failed, due to problems of bringing the various social sciences together. However, soon afterwards the Bureau of Public Roads began to experience complications in putting some legislation through Congress. The Academy was faced with a practical problem, namely how to participate at a level of local planning in order to overcome these difficulties. Powerful pressures from Congress, the executive, and other bodies reinforced Bronk's initiative to unify the social sciences, which now succeeded. The crucial question was not that of a choice between centralization or decentralization for its own sake, but rather what practical purpose would be served by centralization. Further examples of the effect of such external forces are found in the current focus on ecology and the environmental problem, together with efforts such as the International Biological Programme, which was important in bringing the various strands of ecology together. Thus, when external pressures are lacking there is little incentive for the social sciences to become centralized; but centralization may follow from practical and concrete needs.

Professor Jolles raised a wider issue. Initially the question had been the dichotomy between centralism and pluralism, and the possibility of learning from the Polish experience. Now there appeared to be agreement that this was a false dichotomy and that the real problem was how to handle the pluralism between scientists everywhere. Following Suchodolski, such problems can only be solved within each country's intellectual and scientific tradition, as well as within its decision-making structure, and this has significant implications with regard to generalized schemata for research organizations similar to those discussed earlier in the conference (cf. Trist, pp. 101–38 above).

Henning Friis considered that Suchodolski's paper outlined one interesting new development; namely, the efforts to relate research to possible changes in society and to focus attention on the problem of identifying the most important changes (i.e. the setting of priorities). This is occurring in a number of countries, and is forcing social scientists, in many instances for the first time probably, to consider what future problems are the most interesting and the most important. Eric Trist stressed that the current efforts of many of the developing nations to become more mobilized towards the future and towards planning demands co-operation across disciplines, and involves more than economic factors. Social scientists working on studies of planning for development find themselves co-operating across national boundaries, hence linking states in different stages of development.

The importance of national cultural differences was then raised by Professor Groenmann. In Holland sociologists work in many areas of application and are linked with almost every sector of government, a situation which contrasts sharply with the French experience discussed by Henri Mendras. To explain this one has to compare the Dutch tradition and experience with those of the French. Professor Groenmann's own impression is of a significant amount of pressure from the Dutch population directed towards urban and rural planning, which entailed the use of sociology. Much of this demand derived at first from the need to rebuild the Netherlands after wartime destruction, when economic and social planning was needed in all domains. Sociology came in through the belief that the main Dutch resource was its population and that demography held the key to estimation of its size and hence to its mobilization. In addition, the Netherlands' battle with the sea for land inspired a tradition of study of human geography which had developed into sociography, a form of descriptive sociology.

Dietrich Goldschmidt rejected mono-causal explanations for complex problems. While there are parallels in the development of the social sciences in different cultures, unique historical reasons account for their differences. The German tradition was broken in the period 1933–45, and although a new sociology developed in this period its impact on politics and on general social life was comparatively small. In post-war Germany sociology recreated itself as an academic discipline with the pre-1933 focus on ideology. Thus it was not generally linked with problems and its contribution to substantive areas was restricted to the fields of education and the labour market. Sociology as currently developed in German universities is now focusing on methodology and even in Konstanz and other newer institutions, these traditions assert themselves. It would appear (as had been noted by Professor Kredar) that for sociology, at any rate, to tackle societal problems there had to be pressure from external bodies aimed at bringing workers to some common task.

In his concluding remarks, Professor Suchodolski took up again some of the questions he had posed in his introduction. First, the role that the social sciences play in contemporary social life is significant only if the planning of research is directed by an emphasis on societal problems, since in a new or developing society these things matter most. This does not mean focusing too narrowly on economic problems. In Poland, while much effort is concerned with industrialization and associated phenomena, work is flourishing on the sociology of the arts (e.g. the theatre and cinema), and on social aspects of medicine and health. These marginal studies must be linked to the areas in which work is more heavily concentrated to achieve an integrated picture of societal development.

The role of the social sciences is limited by the fact that it is not the social scientists but the lawyers, civil servants, and politicians who make the decisions that determine social reality. Policy-makers have great difficulties in communicating their needs to social scientists and evaluating their expertise. This practical limitation is strongly linked to difficulties in implementing advice received from social scientists. At present, social scientists neither play significant roles in establishing policies for the social life of a nation, nor are they in at the origin of new events or instrumental in shaping new attitudes. It is questionable whether the social sciences can ever lead the internal evolution of a country or whether their role is restricted to that of a witness or an observer. A sociologist may be able to provide an explanation of events, but will his skills enable him to perceive them? For them to play a meaningful role in society, social scientists must come to terms with the limitations of their present knowledge and of their capacities for explanation and prediction.

11 National and international policies for social research

Henning Friis

Problems of emerging states, which are the focus of the field of development studies, have primarily been analysed from an economic viewpoint. Furthermore, development has frequently been approached in Western perspectives in that states are seen to progress towards a 'developed' status as their social, economic, and political institutions draw closer to Western models. Both these assumptions are now severely questioned. Political, social, and educational development are seen as being as significant as economic development, while the manner in which such development is achieved may be shaped by culturally specific factors. In a similar manner, aid programmes for developing nations have focused on the natural sciences and technology to the exclusion of the social sciences, while the few attempts that have been made to develop a social science capacity in new states have shown a strong predilection for introducing methodologies and institutional forms purely on the grounds that these have been successful in more advanced contexts.

Henning Friis deals with these problems in this chapter, drawing illustrations from a recent UNESCO Round Table Conference attended by social scientists from both developing and developed countries. Friis underlines the importance of political and ideological issues to the function and development of the social sciences, and draws attention to the possible political implications of social research, a factor that has caused tensions in Latin America and Japan. New approaches to research allocation and institution-building for the social sciences in developing countries are argued for, in particular ones that emphasize the importance of indigenous material, and regional concentration of facilities. Only through these will social scientists in developing countries look inward at the crucial problems of their own region.

Henning Friis is executive director of the Danish National Institute of Social Research in Copenhagen and vice-chairman of the Danish Social Science Council. Chairman of the OECD Committee for scientific and technical personnel, 1958–65, and UN adviser to Ireland and India on applied social research, Professor Friis is author of several works on policy and research, including 'Development of Social Research in Ireland' (1965), 'Social Policy and Social Research in India' (1968).

The increasing national and international interest in the topic of science policy and organization has only recently begun to encompass the social sciences. While several countries, advanced and less advanced, have accepted the need for planned development of the natural and technological sciences, the social sciences have usually not been included in national science policies or else they have a place on the fringe. The result has been that in a period of overall increase in resources for scientific research, resources for the social sciences have fallen behind and are, by any measure, very meagre and scattered in most countries. Lack of support for the social sciences is also reflected at the international level, since aid to social science activities through international and regional organizations is small.

The state of the social sciences is of particular relevance to countries that are endeavouring to enhance their economic and social conditions, as these have immense need for hard facts and theoretical models on which to base development policies and evaluate results. The growth in resources for social research is, however, very slow, and the gap in those resources between developed and less developed countries is rapidly widening.

A UNESCO Round Table on Social Research Policy and Organization was held in Denmark in September 1969, with the objective of discussing policies for social research, with particular emphasis on the needs of developing countries. The key points of the discussions of the Round Table are summarized below. They are of particular importance in any deliberations on social science policy concerned with the problems of the developing nations.[1]

THE ROLES OF SOCIAL RESEARCH IN A TIME OF CHANGE

One major topic that ran through the discussions of the Round Table was the extreme relevance of political and ideological issues to the functions and development of the social sciences. On one hand they determine the relative weight that social scientists in various regions of the world give to the scientific, the technical (applied), and the critical (general educational) roles of their profession. On the other hand political and ideological factors influence the attitude of the public and the decision-makers towards the social sciences.

There are apparent differences between the social science disciplines. Economists are producing 'hard facts', which are accepted as relevant to government planning, and are acting more often in advisory capacities.

Other social scientists often deal with social problems which, in many countries, are not central to government concern. Whether they want it or not, sociologists and psychologists are generally outside the planning process. When they leave their scientific role they tend to be more outspokenly critical and to adopt more utopian viewpoints than is usual among economists. As was said by a participant from the USA: 'Social scientists in government must choose between being influential, maintaining public silence on points of disagreement or being out-spoken, exhibiting their professional honesty at the cost of their political entrée. Only the court jester is permitted to mock the king.'

A lack of popularity of social sciences among decision-makers is a feature in many countries, either because the scientists are criticizing government or because they deal with matters that are looked upon as esoteric to those grappling with the pressing problems facing their country.

This is particularly true in Latin America where tension due to the political implications of social research has been increasing in intensity during the last years. Social scientists prefer to play an intellectual and critical role rather than a technical one. As a Latin American participant stated: 'Their task consists not only in maximizing production within the *status quo*, but in the alteration of the *status quo*, as they cannot imagine modernization without fundamental changes in the basic structure.'

Another Latin American member of the Round Table foresaw that 'the economic, political, and demographic crisis of the underdeveloped countries will limit liberty of research and diminish the resources for development research', but also that there are opposite trends that promote research, such as an increasing number of social scientists and the view that 'in influential circles of world opinion it is considered that the development of the poor and dependent countries cannot be carried out without large structural reforms'.

In Japan there have been many cases of co-operation between social scientists and big business, but there has been a great deal of controversy with respect to this collaboration, and many scientists tend to be aloof in their attitude towards 'the establishment' or to take a critical role.

Several other participants, from developed as well as less developed countries, found within their countries an increasing interest in a closer relation between the social scientists and policy-making bodies. Eric Trist has pointed to the new relationship between science and society that has led to the emergence of domain-based, problem-oriented research with the involvement of scientists, professionals, administrators, and political representatives. 'The texture of their relationships differs from what is fundamental research where scientists' interest dominate, or applied research where user-interest dominates. The relations of the different types of actor in a problem-oriented domain are that of collaboration' (Trist, 1970).

In most countries the efforts to promote social research that can be useful for policy formation have hitherto shown rather meagre results, except in the field of applied economics. The reason is partly that existing research usually has not been relevant to actual situations, partly that it has not been presented in a way that has made its implications understandable for policy-makers and administrators. Generally the prospective consumers, for their part, have not shown serious interest in using research results even where these might be relevant to their work; demand has been limited and the absorptive capacity for existing research has been small.

On the topic of the relationship between researchers and users, it would appear that if social research is to be of greater use to planning in the future, more understanding of the nature and significance of policy-oriented research must be developed in governments as well as in the academic community.

The Round Table pointed to the need for professionals inside administrative and planning bodies who could become gate-keepers of the client-researcher relationship. These middle-men should provide channels of diffusion for externally generated knowledge and be able to identify relevant research problems within the system. In order to increase the absorptive capacity for social research results it would be necessary to teach planners and administrators social science and the use of the social sciences. The social scientists must on their part be more skilled in the transfer process from research to application (Cherns, 1970).

POLICIES FOR SOCIAL RESEARCH

Resources

Competent social science capability in most countries is a scarce resource and exists mainly in some of the most developed societies. The problem of lack of trained personnel for social research is not only a problem of quantity, but in many countries also of quality. One serious deficiency, particularly in developing countries, is that most graduates have inadequate training and experience in the theoretical and practical aspects of social research work. Some university departments are aware of this problem, but it would be useful if more university departments in the various social science disciplines included not only the theoretical aspects of research methodology in their curriculum, but also practical exercises.

Indigenous teaching material for this purpose is lacking in most developing countries. There is, for instance, no source book or analysis of problems related to the preparation of questionnaires and interviewing in India, although much energy has been spent on sampling techniques. Teaching on other important aspects of survey research, therefore, is based on American and English textbooks, which are insufficient guides for research in India.

A problem common in most countries is the scarcity of skilled specialists in theoretical statistics and programming and other fields that support empirical research.

Most research institutions have insufficient technical research facilities. This is a particular handicap in empirical research, which requires an administrative and technical apparatus for sampling, interviewing, and data-processing. Only a few countries have an organization for sample surveys and computer services available to social researchers. As long as the services of national survey research units are not available one method of obtaining comparable nationwide data is to initiate co-operation between qualified research institutions in the various regions of the country.

There is in most developing countries an extreme scarcity of national funds for social research and the funds that are available are insufficient to meet the costs of modern empirical social research.

In this period of scarcity of funds and trained personnel, social research in many developing countries has been organized by foreign social scientists and supported by funds from foreign countries. Initially this has been necessary and helpful. However, there are political and scientific problems that are often attached to reliance on bilateral aid to the social sciences. In its final report on International Co-operation in the Development of Social Science Research the participants of the Round Table expressed their view on foreign aid in the following way: 'On account of the obvious policy implications of many social research findings, the exclusion of local scientists from the design, execution, and control of research projects is undesirable from a scientific point of view and fraught with potential political danger.'

It was felt that social science research under the control of outsiders tended to serve the latter's own biases or ends and the academic traditions from which they came. This 'control' was seen as not conducive to the natural growth of new theories and to the needs of the area or nation, or to the general healthy growth of the profession.

Economists and statisticians, more particularly, in some developing countries use resources of other countries bilaterally to mutual benefit.

The use, however, of regional centres of international bodies to design or conduct research in areas of social science scarcity would be preferable to unequal bilateral ventures.

One considerable difficulty in social research in most countries – developed as well as less developed – is the lack of stable financing for continued research programmes. Almost all projects are financed on a project to project basis.

Ad hoc financing of research undertakings makes it difficult to undertake long-run planning of research programmes, and often necessitates a research institute's accepting projects to which it would otherwise give a lower priority. Where a continual flow of projects is not assured, the institution may be forced to dismiss good staff members, whereby experiences gained through earlier research are lost for the institution. It is also time-consuming to hunt and wait for money, and the grants do not usually cover indirect management costs.

To avoid these difficulties it is important to establish some stable research institutions with a permanent or semi-permanent basic budget. Wherever additional grants for specific projects are obtained, necessary funds for overhead costs must be included.

It is paradoxical that in a situation of scarcity of funds and manpower for social research, social science throughout the world has been characterized by a scattering of resources.

Even in small countries social research takes place at a considerable number of institutions, which usually work without much co-operation. The research institutes are, as a rule, rather small in size. This is the case not only in less developed countries, but also in countries with greater resources.

It can be argued that when possibilities of working as a social scientist are not limited to a few institutions, greater possibilities exist for absorbing scientists who are diverse in quality and in orientation. Particularly in a period where political powers curtail the work of social scientists, excessive concentration of activities in a few institutions is a dangerous strategy, while pluralization of centres of activity is a way out of possible breakdown of one or more of them (Cornblit, 1970).

While this position may be acceptable in a period of crisis, the author forwarded the view that for empirical social research to be able to use modern methodology and techniques, a certain concentration of researchers in larger units is necessary. Furthermore many types of social research and in particular problem-oriented research usually requires a group of researchers representing several disciplines. In such cases it is preferable that the institution has more than one or two representatives of the various disciplines, as they tend to be professionally isolated if their number is too small.

Taken together these various factors lead to the conclusion that at least some social research institutes in each country must be increased to a far larger size than is now generally the case.

In its final report the Round Table stated the view that

> The time has come to increase decisively the scale of resources provided for the social sciences and also to achieve greater concentration of effort. The discussions made clear that if research capability is to be effective, resources should be assembled into minimum size critical masses. More specifically figures quoted from various sources would suggest a small-size institution for empirical research of 30 to 40 professionals with a continuing annual operating budget of around $250,000 to medium-sized institutions of 70 to 100 professionals with budgets around $1,000,000. The physical plant, library facilities, access to computing services, adequate clerical help and similar factors are the basic necessities to make such an institution viable.

Development Policies

The Round Table report proposed the following national development policy for social science research:

> The first priority is clearly the establishment of a number of viable multi-disciplinary social science research institutions, capable not only of doing research but also of training social scientists at all levels and servicing other social science institutions. The standards of research and training of such an institution should be at the highest international level. In fact these centres should be the foci for the growth of high quality social science. The staff should represent the entire range of social science disciplines; there should be library facilities, computer facilities, clerical services and other duplicating and mechanical devices, now considered basic to a modern research institution.
>
> The training of an adequate body of highly competent social science professionals and the continued production of a large enough well-trained body of professionals are the *sine-qua-non* of social science development. In order to reach the level of self-generating growth the minimum critical mass of social scientists must be trained. Further, various strategies, adapted to the conditions existing in different parts of the world, need to be developed for this purpose, for example making working conditions and local salaries attractive. A local multi-disciplinary research institution as described above would be the best long-term solution for providing scientific manpower as it would be using locally developed theory, locally provided training materials, local field conditions for research and have a far lower rate of brain drain.

The scattering of research resources is due not only to lack of institutional concentration, but also to the absence in most countries, socialist as well as liberal, of policies leading to systematic planning of social research activities. The individualism of the academics and the lack of interest of governments have contributed to scientific anarchy. In all countries it is apparent that on crucial areas and problems basic information is non-existent, or much of the available research is out of date. Even where numerous studies on related problems have been or are being carried out in the country, usually in small geographical areas, little co-ordination has been accomplished. The most serious problem is not so much overlapping of research efforts, but rather a lack of basic common thinking and co-operation which could improve the quality of research and enhance the possibilities for accumulation of knowledge.

A limited number of countries have established National Social Science Councils or similar bodies, which have among their objectives the formulation of policies for development of the social sciences in their country. All have initiated closer collaboration between social scientists inside disciplines as well as between disciplines. Some of them have investigated the situation and the needs of the social sciences and are mapping out strategies for research and research collaboration in areas where there are serious gaps. A few councils are in the process of promoting the improvement of the general infrastructure of the social sciences, such as documentation centres and data archives. Many distribute grants for post-graduate studies and act as government research foundations for the social sciences, which enhances their possibility for directing the social sciences.

Several participants of the Round Table considered that the need to establish National Social Science Councils was immediate, in order that policies for development of the social sciences in their countries would be formulated and to promote government commitment to such policies. The councils should also play the roles of clearing-house and co-ordinator for research projects presented by the various research units, including those located in ministries and foreign research bodies.

Organizational Problems

The Round Table not only studied the broad policy problems of the social sciences, but also dealt with such organizational problems of social science institutions as training of staff, job satisfaction, and internal communication (Campbell, 1970).

The need for staff training as a continuing process was emphasized, including briefing of new staff members, continual staff seminars on methodological and substantive problems, and discussion of research plans and finished reports for diffusion of experiences. Non-scientific staff should also receive training in order that they can relieve the researchers of technical work.

One major obstacle to research in university institutions in many countries is the heavy teaching load and the low salaries of university teachers, which drive them to take on extra outside teaching and other such income-giving activities.

Several methods of improving this situation were mentioned, ranging from an increase in salary for university teachers who concentrate on research to the establishment of special research units inside the university structure, or of autonomous institutes. An intermediate arrangement is found in some countries, where staff members of autonomous research institutes are permitted to teach for a limited number of hours at a university. This arrangement ascertains that research is their main job, but that they keep in touch with colleagues outside their institute and give students the benefit of their research experience.

INTERNATIONAL CO-OPERATION IN THE DEVELOPMENT OF SOCIAL RESEARCH

As was mentioned earlier, social research in developing countries has been dominated by foreign influence. This influence has not only been exerted through control of funds. 'Western' research problems, theories, and methods have to a great extent been taken over by social scientists in other parts of the world, and have not been tested or questioned sufficiently. Even inadequate research has indicated that the unintelligent application of 'Western' models has not been very fruitful. New models are required, and there is now a need for a new orientation: for social scientists in developing countries to look inward to the crucial problems of their own region:

> Whereas most social scientists have hitherto had their particular world-wide disciplines as their principal frame of reference, they should now rather utilize their pooled interdependence for the study of the national, cultural and economic regions. This would both assist the development of such regions and provide a context for new theoretical orientations. Depending on the size of the country or the region, an orientation to that area or region, a pooling of manpower and other resources would in the long run pay the best dividends. Sometimes, where critical shortages of trained personnel, computer facilities, or money exist, international co-operation may be used in politically acceptable mixes consistent with the ultimate end – the development of a viable social science research capability useful for that area.

The Round Table's report suggested several mechanisms to facilitate a higher degree of regional communication between social scientists. Co-ordinated research in problem-oriented areas would bring small groups of scientists into meaningful communication. Larger regional meetings on problem-oriented areas, agricultural development, urbanization, population policies, etc., would be another method. A special social science publication for a region would help communication. Exchange of staff on specific projects or teaching assignments could bring about a meaningful communication between scientists.

It was also proposed that a common technical centre be available in each region, by which smaller countries in particular could be assisted:

> The development of at least one regional social science documentation centre, computer centre and data bank in each region of the world, functionally articulated with other national centres of the region, is called for in this second decade of development. This triple effort would call for fairly large resource allocations, but would have a demonstration effect and greatly enhance the national and regional utility of the social sciences in the next decade. Hence these centres would need to be future-oriented, adequately staffed and financed, and have a large flexible capacity for expansion in various needed areas.

The Round Table emphasized that in the Second Development Decade it would be necessary to give the social sciences a central place in international assistance programmes as a prerequisite for development planning. It found that the activities in this field by UNESCO and other international bodies have hitherto been marginal and scattered.

Whatever the reasons are for the low priority that international organizations until now have given to expansion of national and regional resources for social research in developing countries, the time is now ripe for a forceful action. It is my conviction that funds from the United Nations Development Programme and the International Bank for Reconstruction and Development along with concerted actions from the Specialized Agencies and the UN Regional Commissions should be directed towards maximum support for institution-building for social research on a big scale.

Let me conclude with one more quotation from the report of the Round Table on Social Research Policy and Organization:

> The decade has also seen some excellent research and the development by leaps and bounds of methodological sophistication in the social sciences. In fact social science today stands at the threshold of great expectations. Computer technology and the formal and empirical

methods which are now being diffused into all the social sciences have re-oriented the entire spectrum of social science disciplines and given them an integrated impact which no single discipline could formerly make. The social sciences are thus becoming more operational and playing an increasingly important role in the application of science and technology. We foresee that the needs for social science are going to escalate as they become integrated into a total scientific system applicable to the modernization of man.

Note

[1] The Conference was organized by the Danish Government as a part of its special contribution to the United Nations Development programme and with the assistance of the Danish National Institute of Social Research. Twenty-six leading social scientists from Africa, Asia, Latin America, USA, USSR, and Western Europe participated in the Round Table.

References

CAMPBELL, A., Problems of Staff Development in Social Research Organizations. *International Social Science Journal* **22**, 2, pp. 214–25, 1970.

CHERNS, A. B., Relations between Research in Institutions and Users of Research. *International Social Science Journal* **22**, 2, pp. 226–42, 1970.

CORNBLIT, O., Factors affecting Scientific Productivity: the Latin American Case. *International Social Science Journal* **22**, 2, pp. 243–63, 1970.

FRIIS, H., Development of Social Research in Ireland. *Institute of Public Administration* **65**, 1965.

— Social Policy and Social Research in India. India International Centre, New Delhi, 1968.

TRIST, E., Social Research Institutions: Styles, Structures, Scale. *International Social Science Journal* **22**, 2, pp. 301–26, 1970.

Interchapter

The major points arising out of the discussion of Professor Friis's paper are concerned with the issues of institution-building in the social sciences within developing countries; linked to this is the desirability of regional concentration of research and research facilities.

One American participant wondered if the Round Table had not 'given up too soon' by stressing regional development. Social science, he considered, is unfortunately all too often culture-bound and the design of institutions along the lines of imperfect Western models might improve this situation by widening perspectives and refining models that were at present in use.

However, the general consensus of the discussion was that, taking account of cultural constraints and needs and in particular of limited resource availability, regional concentration of facilities is frequently the optimum policy. Einar Thorsrud reviewed the Scandinavian situation. In this instance resources are so scarce that studies in many areas are in danger of disappearing unless they are conceived on Nordic lines. This policy makes sense because there is a Nordic culture, which is reciprocally reinforced by co-operative action on a regional basis.

Another point of view is that we are being too restrictive in considering regional concentration and development only in connection with the developing nations. Similar problems can be seen within US academic institutions over the last twenty to twenty-five years, especially where institutions have attempted to compete with one another over the development of new courses. In these instances, the problem of scarcity of resources, particularly of manpower, has raised its head all too frequently, and institutions aiming for across-the-board excellence in every department are unable to obtain it. Thus the question arises as to whether, within a particular cultural context, institutions should aim for excellence on a wide scale in many branches of the social sciences or whether they should concentrate on fields of strength for future development.

Speaking in support of regional development, Eric Trist recalled that his own impression from the Copenhagen Round Table conference was that social scientists from the developing areas undoubtedly needed to work within the texture of their own societies and hence become equipped with the use of scientific methods so that they could obtain their own data which was desperately needed. People from the outside could help as sources of external resources but it is doubtful if they could do more than that, since scientists from these countries view processes such as development in totally different terms from those used by Western economists and sociologists.

Replying to these comments, Henning Friis did not see the issue of regional concentration as a major outcome of the Round Table. The emphasis was rather on institution-building and the building of stable infrastructures for the social sciences. Granted this emphasis, the regional aspect comes in only because resources in several countries, particularly the Asian and African nations, are so scarce that some kind of regionalization, at least initially, would be helpful. The issues of Western models and crossnational testing are important but also fraught with danger if they turn interest away from the national to the international community. While crossnational research in the Western area (e.g. US, UK, France, etc.) is moderately successful, many of those coming from India, for example, are little short of disastrous, using in one culture questionnaires designed for another. As a consequence, some of these countries are now turning against foreign social scientists, and foreign workers are either prohibited or required to demonstrate the practical results of their work to the government before leaving the country.

When we talk of concentration of resources into fields of strength, we are dealing with two different things. First, we face the simple lack of basic data that both institutes and individuals (such as survey researchers) require. This is a fundamental need, and a capacity to meet it should be established in all countries not only for general educational purposes and for local knowledge but also for policy and planning. The second issue arises where people wish to develop a certain area or discipline to a high level of competence (possibly one of international recognition); in situations where resources are scarce, the only solution lies in concentration. However, these issues should be separated and the first is of higher importance.

An economist then confessed as to being a little uneasy as regards both the direction of the discussion and the thrust of the paper. What people seemed to be advocating almost without exception was that the social sciences had a particular cost-effectiveness for the developing nations who should consequently devote more of their limited resources to the advance of these areas. Such a line is dangerous, since at present there are serious problems in applying knowledge in the social sciences. One must avoid suggesting that investment in the social sciences will be *ipso facto* beneficial. We do not really know how to ensure application and indeed we do know that application is often difficult for political reasons. More generally we are as yet unable to apply a principle of verifiability to our research results.

Henning Friis reacted sharply to this challenge. He was in complete disagreement with such arguments and pointed out that the Copenhagen meeting had been particularly concerned with a country's capacity to absorb research results. This issue was in fact discussed at Copenhagen by a delegate from Tunisia, who pointed to two types of research that seemed badly needed: first, short-term basic knowledge, which could be utilized in planning, and, second, more long-range research (e.g. model-building) which would not have an immediate input into the planning machinery but which was nevertheless necessary to mould the minds of policy-makers in the future. Utilization is indeed a problem, but it can in part be bridged by the recruitment of good social scientists into political and administrative posts; this is already happening in Africa, where the movement of trained manpower into administrative cadres can be attributed to the appearance of strong institutions such as the Nigerian Institute of Economic and Social Research. However, in Asia (apart from India) and in Latin America, the situation is somewhat different, especially in the latter case where, although there is a relatively large output of excellent social scientists, these are very far removed from the actual policy-influencing process.

Supporting Henning Friis, Albert Cherns observed that philosophic doubts of the type earlier expressed in relation to cost-effectiveness had not been put forward at the Copenhagen conference by delegates from the developing countries, but rather by people from the 'effete' West. The former had, in fact, no doubt about the potential and the utility of social science, and possibly one reason for this difference in perspective was that they were hard up against the problems of trying to develop.

12 Social science meta-policy

Some concepts and applications

Yehezkel Dror

Studies of policies for the social sciences, and of means of involving social science knowledge in policy-making, implicitly (if not explicitly) involve a prescriptive element in that they seek means of achieving better policy-making or greater utilization. In this way they deal with elements of the policy sciences, an interdiscipline that attempts to understand how policies are actually made at a variety of levels and within different cultural contexts, and through such an understanding how these policies can be improved.

Yehezkel Dror, a leading advocate of the policy sciences, has introduced the term meta-policy (briefly, a policy on the making of policies) which may be used descriptively to explain past policy-making behaviour and to improve knowledge on policy-making by providing models to interrelate policy variables, and prescriptively to suggest structural and institutional arrangements necessary for better policy-making. In this chapter, he briefly examines how the meta-policy concept may be applied to the social science policy area and, in particular, what prescriptive guides it gives with regard to personnel, organizational structures, policy-making inputs, and policy-making methods which may be required for more optimal and efficient social science policy-making.

At present Professor of Public Administration at the Hebrew University of Jerusalem, Professor Dror has recently been attached to the Rand Corporation, Santa Monica, California, and to Rand, New York, as a senior research fellow. His publications and activities have been directed towards the development of concepts and tools in the policy sciences and their application to concrete social issues and strategic problems. Many of his ideas are set out in his book *Public Policymaking Re-examined* (1968).

INTRODUCTION

The main purpose of this brief and exploratory paper is to present a frame of appreciation and some concepts, which may help in the formulation of some social science policy issues and their examination. To sharpen the ideas, this paper is presented in 'outline' form – without elaboration, detailed consideration, and operationalized applications. Intellectually, this paper is based on theoretic work on the improvement of policy-making, on the integration of social science into policy-making, and on relations between social science and analytical decision approaches. Empirically and experimentally, this paper is based on some surveys of applied social science endeavours and on participant observation in policy research, which try to fuse social science into policy analysis.

I use the term 'meta-policy' to refer to policies on how to make policies. Meta-policies deal (i) with the characteristics of the policy-making system, including structure, process patterns, personnel, inputs, and stipulated outputs; and (ii) with master policies (or 'mega-policies'), which include strategies, overall goals, basic assumptions, conceptual frameworks, policy instruments, and similar interpolicy directives.

The concept of meta-policy can be used behaviourally, to describe and explain actual (past, present, and expected future) phenomena. A meta-policy behavioural analysis can improve our knowledge on actual policy-making by providing better frameworks for identifying and ordering data and improved models for interrelating policy variables. The concept of meta-policy can also be used normatively, to indicate meta-policy arrangements needed for better policy-making. These two main uses of a meta-policy framework are interrelated, in the sense that all normative recommendations must be based, in part, on behavioural knowledge; and that collection of behavioural information depends, in part, on the uses of that information in which we are interested. Therefore, meaningful and reliable application of the meta-policy concept to social science requires comprehensive knowledge on actual social science meta-policies, on relations between social science meta-policies and social science outputs, and on the values that we want social science to advance (including knowledge for its own sake). One of the main uses of the concept of social science meta-policy should be to stimulate research, study, contemplation, design, and analysis focusing explicitly on the meta-policy level.

META-POLICY AND SOCIAL SCIENCE POLICY

To illustrate the applications of the meta-policy concept to social science policy, I will take up a few main meta-policy issues, explain them in short, and transform the general meta-policy issues into social science meta-policy issues. I will use normative language, but the same issues can easily be transformed into behavioural ones:

Short explanation of issue	*Transformation into social science meta-policy issue*
A. BASIC MODUS OPERANDI OF POLICY-MAKING SYSTEMS	
Mix between market, polycentric, and hierarchic structures in policy-making systems, with spontaneous evolution of policy as one extreme.	How far should there be 'social science policy' involving explicit policy-making and a formalized policy-making system? What should be the basic *modus operandi* of that system, varying from 'control by overlapping peer groups' to central decision-making.
B. MAIN COMPONENTS OF POLICY-MAKING SYSTEM, ESPECIALLY (A) ORGANIZATIONS, AND (B) PERSONNEL	
What should the main components of the policy-making system be, with special attention to (a) organizational components, and (b) policy-making personnel? In addition to usual components, the possibilities of new types of organizations (such as policy research organizations) and new types of professionals (e.g. policy analysts) raise novel opportunities and issues.	What special organizations for social science policy-making should be developed? With what functions, power, and resources? For instance, what about permanent social science policy analysis units? What should the social science policy-making personnel be? What about participation of politicians, administrators, and community representatives in various social science policy-making roles? What about training of professionals who specialize in issues of social science policy?
C. INFORMATION INPUTS INTO POLICY-MAKING	
What types of information are needed for good policy-making? Which parts of that information are cost-effective? What arrangements are needed to collect and process that information and for introducing it into actual policy-making?	The general problems of information for better policy-making apply directly to social science policy. Specific information needs include, for instance, data on current studies and manpower, data on image of social science held by various relevant groups, feedback on results of study – both theoretic and applied. Criteria to ascertain results and standards for appraising them are also needed.
D. MAIN POLICY-MAKING METHODS	
Patterning of policy-making, phasing in time-stream (e.g. by sequential decision-making) and development of methods and techniques for explicit analysis (e.g. policy analysis, benefit-cost estimation, multiple-year planning, etc.).	Development of methods for social science policy-making, on different macro-levels (international, crossnational, national) and micro-levels (e.g. universities, institutes, etc.). Policy analysis and sequential decision-making seem especially applicable, but research explicitly directed at developing methods for social science policy-making seems urgently needed.

Short explanation of issue	*Transformation into social science meta-policy issue*
E. MAIN MEGA-POLICIES IN PARTICULAR ON	
(a) Values and cutting-off horizons (including the question, how far values and cutting-off horizons should be explicated?)	
Master policies guiding policy-making on specific issues, in particular on: the main values at which policy-making should aim, with explicit determination of considered impact-space and of borders of alternative sets to be considered. The costs (political, psychological, moral, etc.) of classifying values and cutting-off horizons must be considered to decide how far to proceed with this mega-policy.	Master policies guiding policy-making on social science policy, in particular on: the values at which social science policy should be oriented, such as (1) pure knowledge, and (2) social goals specific and/or as set down by legitimate policy-makers. The borders of 'social science policy' – what are social sciences, and how far should social science policy be considered as a component of broader issues (e.g. social policy as a whole)? What are the limits of values and issues to be considered as subjects for social science policy? What are the costs of establishing this mega-policy and what are its benefits (including value sensitivity analysis – does this mega-policy really make much difference)?
(b) Nature of operational goals	
Should policies be mainly directed at achieving specific goals, to provide options, or to build up resources for the future?	Should social science policies be directed at solving defined theoretic or applied questions? And/or provide knowledge that can be used to deal with various questions? And/or build up the resources to develop knowledge in the future (through training of academic and applied scientists, longitudinal data-collection, refinement of methodology, etc.)?
(c) Degrees of innovation	
Incremental change *vs.* radical change; how far to encourage 'heresy' and far-reaching innovations, and in what way.	How far should social science policy aim at incremental progress and/or at radical breakthroughs – up to 'scientific revolutions'? How to encourage/control far-reaching innovation – what about incentives, resources allocation, peer support for unconventional approaches?
(d) Attitudes to risks (this is closely related to point (c) above)	
Mix between maximax, minimax, etc.	How far should social science policy become adventurous, follow risky research possibilities (e.g. on altered states of consciousness), take up taboo issues (e.g. as tried in the Chicago jury studies), and provide low reliability recommendations?

Short explanation of issue	*Transformation into social science meta-policy issue*
	(e) Time preferences
Preference between outputs located on different points of the time stream.	Should social science policy be more oriented to immediate issues and problems (as expressed, for instance, by the social advocacy approach) or adopt longer (how long?) time preferences?

As already indicated, this is too schematic a presentation, the obvious preference being for some mix between various policy-making system alternatives and mega-policy alternatives. But the concept 'mix' – however in accord with our *a priori* preferences for some 'golden mean' – is of little help. The question is 'what mix?' Explicit considerations of social science meta-policy issues hopefully can help at least in formulating relevant questions, and thereby taking one step in the direction of identification of preferable meta-policy mixes.

AN ILLUSTRATION OF META-POLICY IN USE

To illustrate further the uses of the meta-policy concept, let me indicate in short the implications for social science meta-policy of one view of a desired direction for the development of social science, namely the view that social sciences should, in part, fuse with analytical decision approaches and serve as a foundation for policy sciences. Let me just emphasize that (a) here this proposal is used only as an illustration to 'exercise' the meta-policy concept, and (b) in any case, the proposal aims to add an approach to social science policy, without in any way degrading the importance of other approaches.

I will proceed by referring to the various meta-policy issues by the numbers used above and indicate the respective meta-policy implications of the proposed approach (which, strictly speaking, belongs itself to social science mega-policy):

A. Explicit social science policy-making is needed, in order to advance efforts to move in the policy sciences direction. Much of this policy-making can proceed in 'invisible colleges', but some formalization seems to be required. This is needed especially to get co-operation between the interested scholars and institutions, and assure at least minimum support by the social science community as a whole.

B (a). Special organizations which critically consider social science policy may be needed to perceive the need for change in the direction of policy sciences. *Ad hoc* committees can (and do) fulfil important functions in this direction. Specific social science policy units are also necessary to support the efforts, supervise them (to avoid the fate, for instance, of studies that get ruined through over-popularization) and advance them.

B (b). The special characteristics of policy sciences require more heterogeneous personnel than 'normal' social science policy-making. In particular, an interdisciplinary composition is needed, with some participation also of policy practitioners – politicians as well as senior executives.

C. Information on persons able and willing to participate in a policy sciences development effort, on relevant studies and on relevant experience is needed. As much of the relevant personnel, material, and experience is located outside the 'normal' social science community (e.g. at policy research organizations, legislative and governmental research units, and private consultants), a suitable information network must be built up.

D. Sequential decision-making on an international scale seems a preferable method.

E (a). The values of policy sciences are mainly instrumental-normative policy-making improvement, within the boundaries of morally acceptable policy goals. The boundaries of policy-making here are much broader than in 'normal' social science policy, including other disciplines and some aspects of politics as well.

E (b). A main initial operational goal must be to start and build up the infrastructure of policy sciences, including: establishment and reinforcement of policy sciences research organizations; establishment and reinforcement of policy sciences teaching; initiation of suitable professional activities, such as periodicals, conferences, etc.; and, last but not least, recruitment of financial support. In other words, a main mega-policy should be to build up resources for building up policy sciences.

E (c). Very innovative oriented, with presumption of designing a 'scientific revolution'.

E (d). Significant propensity to accept risks.

E (e). Preference for intermediate future, about five years and more ahead, with main results to take much longer.

My overall conclusion and recommendation is that every concern with social science policy should devote considerable attention to explicit consideration of social science meta-policy issues.

BIBLIOGRAPHIC NOTE

To compensate somewhat for the brevity of this paper, let me refer the interested reader to some of my writings in which ideas presented in this paper are discussed at greater length.

The concept of meta-policy and its relations to policy-making are developed at length in *Public Policymaking Re-examined.* Some additional meta-policy concepts are discussed in 'Policy Analysis: A Theoretic Framework and Some Basic Concepts'.

A few empiric findings illustrating the situation which, in my opinion, make necessary some fusion between parts of applied social science and analytical decision approaches are presented in 'The Uses of Sociology in Public Administration: Four Cases from Israel and The Netherlands', in Lazarsfeld *et al.* (1967, pp. 418–26). The proposal to move in the direction of fusion between parts of applied social science and analytical decision approaches and to advance together towards policy sciences is presented in 'Social Sciences and Social Problems: Some Comments on the Paper of Henry W. Riecken'. It is discussed at length in 'Systems Analysis and Applied Social Sciences', in Horowitz (ed., forthcoming).

The idea of policy sciences is presented in 'Prolegomena to Policy Sciences'. The needs for special policy sciences teaching designs are discussed in 'Teaching of Policy Sciences: Design for a Doctorate University Program'.

Finally, a framework for examining some social science policy issues within a broad perspective is proposed in 'A General Systems Approach to Uses of Behavioral Sciences for Better Policymaking'.

References

DROR, Y., The Uses of Sociology in Public Administration: Four Cases from Israel and the Netherlands. In *The Uses of Sociology*, P. Lazarsfeld, W. Sewell and H. Welensky (eds.). Basic Books, New York, 1967.

— *Public Policymaking Re-examined.* Chandler, San Francisco, 1968.

— Systems Analysis and Applied Social Sciences. In *Proceedings of Rutgers University and Trans-Action Magazine Conference on Public Policy and Social Sciences*, Irving L. Horowitz (ed.) (forthcoming). (Earlier version: RAND paper P-4248, November 1969.)

— A General Systems Approach to Uses of Behavioral Sciences for Better Policy-making. In *General Systems Dynamics*, Ernest O. Attinger (ed.). Karger, New York, 1970. (Earlier version: RAND paper P-4091, May 1969.)

— Social Sciences and Social Problems: Some Comments on the Paper of Henry W. Riecken. *Social Science Information* 9, 1, pp. 187–91, February 1970. (Earlier versions: RAND paper P-4202, September 1969.)

— Prolegomena to Policy Sciences. *Policy Sciences* 1, 1, pp. 135–50, Spring, 1970. (Earlier version: RAND paper P-4283.)

— Teaching of Policy Sciences: Design for a Doctorate University Programme. *Social Sciences Information* 9, 2, pp. 101–22, April 1970. (Earlier version: RAND paper P-4128–1.)

— Policy Analysis: A Theoretic Framework and Some Basic Concepts. RAND paper P-4156, July 1969.

Interchapter

In introducing Yehezkel Dror's paper, Dr Geoffrey Roberts emphasized a hope that the paper, or at least some of the arguments contained in it, might provide the basis of an integrative framework around which much of the proceedings of the conference could be related. Turning to the paper itself, he drew attention to Dror's concept of meta-policy, i.e. 'policies on how to make policies', which deals with the characteristics of the policy-making system including structure, process patterns, personnel inputs, and stipulated outputs and with master (or mega-) policies that include strategies, overall goals, and basic assumptions. Meta-policy is a concept that can be descriptive, i.e. it can be an analysis of what policies and arrangements exist, or it can be prescriptive, i.e. it can deal with what arrangements should exist for better policy-making. We should take account of both aspects with regard to social science policy. There is indeed some doubt as to whether a social science policy is either possible or desirable, but despite this Dror correctly draws attention to the need to consider these facts explicitly and not to let them go by default. Social science policy-making requires both an interdisciplinary composition and the constant interaction of practitioners, namely the social scientists and the policy-makers. Dror's paper highlighted the following points:

a framework such as this one is needed to relate the disparate topics of the conference;

a policy for social science is more than simply a question of organizing social science research; it involves also the utilization of social science and the communication of social science findings;

the suggestion in Dr Riecken's paper that people may not want a policy for social science, and that even if they want one, it may be unobtainable, should not preclude attempts to give the matter conscious deliberation rather than giving up at the complexity of the question;

we should not confuse pessimism about this topic (a term that seemed to be used quite frequently) with an ability to identify or to recognize the complexities that are involved.

The discussion that followed welcomed the arguments and style of Professor Dror's paper. In Eric Trist's view it illustrates a method of viewing problems that is growing considerably in many parts of the world. In particular this involves the interaction of administrators and government on a continuous basis and their acceptance of policy-making as a dynamic process without sharp cut-offs.

Professor Wilson, however, was a little more conservative in his reaction. He wondered if Dror had not underplayed the role of politics in the decision-making process and whether a policy-maker reading Dror's paper would not query where politics came in. He would not consider it possible to have a neutral discussion involving both policy-makers and social scientists without examining the large masses of power that were wielded behind the policies concerned. Who then would be considered policy-makers – the politicians and leaders of political parties or a wider spectrum of actors including governmental advisers, administrators, and personnel close to government, e.g. foundation executives?

Answering these points, Geoffrey Roberts stressed that in the first instance Dror would be one of the last people to neglect politics. His analyses have always taken full account of issues such as political feasibility, i.e., that it is not enough to quantify decisions and then to take the best alternative that this indicated. Here Dror is not chiefly concerned with an explicit definition of the policy-makers and their values but rather with structures that would bring social scientists and the policy sector together – structures not for taking decisions but for permitting full discussions.

For Professor Goldschmidt the dichotomy of the social scientist and the policy-maker was a little forced, since the latter is frequently essentially an administrator. He often wondered, at meetings of independent experts and administrators, whether the administrators themselves were not also 'experts', only from different angles. In Germany, the role of the expert is frequently that of a missionary whose objective is to break down some of the administrators' conservatism. However, having done this, the 'expert' withdraws and takes no part in the decision process.

In reply, Dr Roberts agreed that it was essential to take account of cultural backgrounds and that there was indeed little likelihood of one solution universal for all social structures. This is brought out by Dror in both the current paper and his earlier work.

But how in the interaction of the policy sector with social science do the actions of the former depend on their perceptions of the capabilities of the various disciplines and, further, to what extent is the ability of different disciplines to act together in following the same policy related to the extent to which they see each other as relevant? Albert Cherns considered these as important factors in any understanding of the relationship between social science and policy-maker, which needed to be made explicit. One of the things standing out in the current discussions is that a great deal already exists in terms of unobtrusive or non-reactive measures (i.e. one does not have to ask people questions about their images of the social sciences, rather their actions speak for them). If we compare the occasions on which social scientists have been brought in by policy-makers with those on which they have not, we see what kind of policy social science is relevant for, and what kind of social science is relevant to what policies. An illustration of this can be drawn from an examination of development policies. Initially almost solely economic, now development policies reflect the recognition that development is a social, political, and educational issue as well as an economic one. How has this come about? How has this recognition taken place – has the image of the social sciences changed or has the problem changed? Or is there a relationship between how the problem is perceived and the images of the social sciences?

Expanding on the issue of images, Orville Brim raised questions regarding the acceptance of social science policy and also of the relationship between the sciences. Many people in the US view the physical and biological sciences as major obstacles to the acceptance of social science, both in terms of increased funding and in acceptance in the councils of policy – is this a particular US experience or is it shared in other countries? The larger issue, however, is that social science challenges time-honoured assumptions underlying public practice. This is particularly true with regard to the legal and medical professions; however, compared with the natural scientists, the lawyers' opposition was as nothing, since lawyers are not in competition with social scientists for resources, political influence, and positions of power. The images of the social sciences must be viewed separately from the viewpoint of different professions, and in the US indeed the hard sciences may obstruct the development of the social sciences.

One participant then pointed out that the impact of the social sciences on individuals was undoubtedly more personalized and more frightening than that of physical sciences. Shaping people's intrinsic developmentally based view on why people behave the way they do is not teaching to an open mind but to a fragile defensive structure (i.e. one attacked it as one taught). People act so as to minimize disturbances to firmly held concepts; if one looks at the needs for advisers as articulated by government or military bodies, one notes that they seek people who share their basic conceptual scheme. Advice is primarily a means of sanctioning already held views, while seeking it out acts to reassure decision-makers that they are obtaining a full appreciation of their problem.

Dr Jenkins agreed that the social sciences were not neutral. The knowledge and advice they offer clash sharply with the values and positions of the policy-makers. Dror's approach involves the analysis of the policy-making system so that values and assumptions are made explicit; consequently the interaction of policy-maker and adviser can be more easily understood. On a broader issue, the discussions too readily contrasted the social sciences stratified internally, with economics at the head, with the unified strength of the natural sciences. This is a misconception. Differentiation and stratification are visible within the natural sciences and nowhere so clearly as in the nature of their subject matter and associated theory. The methods of the life sciences are not those of the earth sciences, nor can we compare meteorology which deals with multivariable problems with theoretical physics. They display the same type of spectrum as existed within the social sciences, frequently linked with a hierarchy of prestige within and between disciplines. The social and natural sciences are not totally separable in terms of exactness and contributions to knowledge – a fairer distinction is that social sciences tackle problems of such a type that the knowledge they produce tends frequently to be diffuse and inexact.

Dr Roberts returned to the issue of images. Areas such as law and economics may be viewed by the political sector and wider publics as conservative disciplines that tend to maintain the *status quo*. In contrast, sociology may be viewed as a revolutionary social science, political science being allocated a liberal-reformist category. In part this is related to the type of language used – economics in its explanations is familiar to administrators, something that cannot be said with conviction for sociological research or political sciences.

Such a classification may depend, as one discussant was quick to point out, on the stage reached by the fashionable theory of a subject; reductionalist and incremental theories such as those of economics are successful both in academic and wider political terms. Albert Cherns, however, pointed out the importance of examining values in any case of this nature. Economics may well look a conservative discipline if the values of the discipline and of the society are congruent. In contrast, however, anthropology has been for many years viewed as a conservative discipline, since it trades in the same values as the societies it describes. Now, in the same instance, if one had consulted an economist, one would have received revolutionary advice, since the latter's proposals would involve the introduction of a set of values different from that which the society already had. Consequently, the issue is not really one of the discipline being conservative, incrementalist, or revolutionary, but much more a question of the congruence between the values of the discipline and the dominant values of society.

A final point was made by Paul Lazarsfeld, who emphasized the importance of developing a wider understanding of the communication and utilization of social science knowledge. At present he is engaged in a project to study the teaching of sociology in medical schools and here in many ways aspects of the users are different and the study requires the development of different methods of tracing them. As a result of this, and many other instances, he was convinced that what is required is a 'theory of application' in a form that will focus on the problem of the connection between knowledge and policy in the social sciences.

Selective bibliography

Ruth Sinclair and Elisabeth Crawford

INTRODUCTION

The classification used in this bibliography does not follow exactly the topics of the conference but is designed to show the main themes that should be considered in formulating social science policies, at national and international level.

The bibliography does not in any way attempt to be comprehensive. The most obvious constraint has been space, hence it does not include references that are more than 10 years old, nor does it list very well-known materials or articles that are too specific. Examples of the latter are those dealing with the functions of particular research councils and research organizations, and descriptive accounts of the growth and present status of the social sciences, having a parochial or narrowly national orientation. References to these and many other types of materials may be found in the bibliographies listed in section 5.

1. Functions and Roles of the Social Sciences

Most of the literature that could be included in this section concerns the specific roles that social scientists have played or could play in the future. There is little discussion on the more general or, may we say, more fundamental questions of what functions and roles do or should social scientists have. For example, is the role of critic or change agent a valid one for the social scientist? Some of the literature in section 3, however, does discuss the appropriate roles for social scientists in problem-solving.

2. Policies towards the Social Sciences

This section contains literature on various aspects of the development and growth of the social sciences. We have pinpointed the areas of the design of institutions, finance, and manpower as ones that are closely interrelated and could be held to form the basis of policies for the development of the social sciences.

One question that may be asked is 'what kind of research in what kind of organization?' Discussion on this can be found in H. Friis's article (pp. 212–25 above) and 'Eleven contributions to a discussion' written in reply to this (1966, 2.1).

Closely related to this is the form and source of finance for social science research, for example, research institutions with no secure source of finance may have to accept contracts with little or no academic content in order to maintain the employment of research workers. Apart from the general issue of the total amount of finance available for social science research and teaching, consideration is given to other questions: the source of finance; the period for which money is given; the conditions (e.g. limitations on publication) attached to the research monies.

In the area of manpower planning, the crucial factor seems to be to achieve a balance between the output of the educational sector and the demands from user-organizations. One of the first problems to be tackled in this area, as with the financing of social science research, is that of data collection. A start has been made in this area, for example, in Britain the publication by the University Grants Committee of a detailed account of the first employment of all university graduates and in Germany the survey of the employment of sociology graduates (2.3).

Discussion of these topics in relation to social science policy is likely to be at a macro-level. One example of the interrelation between the design of institutions, finance, and manpower at a micro-level, however, is Peter Rossi's article (1964, 2.1).

We have also included in this section documents that report on policy discussions and decisions affecting the social sciences, e.g. Report on the Committee on Social Studies. The OECD report 'Social Science and the Policies of Governments' while not relating to specific policy decisions, discusses quite fully areas that require consideration in drawing up social science policies (2.4).

3. The Use of the Social Sciences in Policy or Planning

This section concerns the application of social science to policy and the relationship between social scientists on the one hand and policy-makers and administrators on the other, at different levels and within different organizations.

The application of the social sciences and the role of the social scientist in problem-solving is a topic of interest and controversy in the social science community. There are those who press for greater use of social science knowledge and research results in policy-making, while others point out the dangers of trying to apply social science findings without sufficient theoretical backing. This dilemma is pointed out in the introduction of *The Uses of Sociology* edited by Lazarsfeld *et al.* (3.0). 'The rapid expansion of sociology both in the numbers of sociologists and in the growth of research, makes its use a matter of special concern, we do not want to create expectations which we cannot fulfil, nor do we want to be excluded from the present surge of interest in scientific activities in this country.'

Another thread running through this section is the relationship between social scientists and policy-makers: their different social and institutional structures; different norms and expectations and 'relatively unstructured exchange process between them' (Archibald, 1968, 3.1). Section 3.1 points to some of the alternative approaches that have been suggested to increase utilization of social science research. For example, the 'pragmatist' model (Lompe, 1968, 3.1), the 'collaborative action-research type relationships' (Trist, 1968, 3.1), and the 'policy analysis systems' approach (Dror, 1968, 3.1).

Section 3.2 discusses issues raised in considering what Lear calls the 'fourth dimension of Government', i.e. in addition to the original three branches of government – legislative, executive, and judicial – there would be an independent evaluative branch designed to relate research to public policy (1968, 3.2).

Section 3.3 considers the use of social scientists and social science knowledge within industrial organizations. Literature in both of the last two sections discusses the relationship between the doers and users of research. In relation to public policy-making, Horowitz's article (1969, 3.3) considers how academics view politicians and how politicians view academics. With respect to industry most of the literature deals with the relationship between the consultant and the client – see, for example, the work of Warren Bennis (1966, 3.3).

4. International Collaboration in the Social Sciences

This section has obvious importance, and the limited amount of material in this area may reflect the limited collaboration that exists, for example, in the formation of international teams of researchers. What little international research is carried out is usually supported by the international bodies.

For scholars interested in studying the social sciences on a crossnational basis many problems exist; the wide variation in the status of the subjects; institutional arrangements for teaching and research; the disciplines and sub-disciplines included and the form and extent of government support and planning in the social sciences. These make the task of comparative research exceedingly difficult but also point to the need for international collaboration in the collection of data on the social sciences.

5. Bibliographies

1. FUNCTIONS AND ROLES OF THE SOCIAL SCIENCES

BOULDING, K., *The Impact of the Social Sciences*, Rutgers University Press, New Brunswick, N.J., 1966.

This book discusses the differences in folk and literary knowledge and in scientific knowledge – difference lies not in their methods but in their complexity. Folk knowledge is sufficient for each to deal with his own social system, but society as a whole is too complex to be dealt with in this way and needs scientific knowledge. Advance in knowledge is a two-part process – new theoretical insights and new methods of measurement. Economics is an advanced and useful social science, mainly because of the information available, whereas the international system is characterized by an information system designed to produce false images. Social science will not be successful in the international sphere until we have more data. Suggests international data station should be set up.

CRICK, B., What is truth in social science? *New Society*, No. 88, pp. 20–1, 4 June 1964.

The author argues that social scientists' preoccupation with proving that social science is a science stems from a desire to eliminate bias from their work. The author feels that some kind of commitment is inevitable in the social sciences. Compares social scientists to lawyers who present evidence and argue for a point of view, and do so clearly and concisely, but do not judge.

DE GRAZIA, ALFRED, The Hatred of the New Social Science, *American Behavioral Scientist* 5, pp. 5–13, October 1961.

The author has entered into a defence against the attacks on the new social science with the aim of illuminating the scope and limits of social science. He divides the actions into four groups: sundry bad habits; the impossibility of a social science; insufficiency of social science to provide for human wishes; undesirability of social science. The author examines these categories to reach an understanding of the types of persons engaged in attack upon social science and then considers some statement of what social science is and what it can offer the world.

2. POLICIES TOWARDS THE SOCIAL SCIENCES

2.0 General writings

2.1 Design of institutions for social science research and training

2.2 The financing of social science research and teaching

2.3 Manpower questions
2.4 Documents relating to the formulation of social science policies in different countries
2.5 Types of decisions affecting social science policies

2.0 General Writings

BEALS, RALPH L., *Politics of Social Research*, Aldine, Chicago, 1969.

The book reports a study undertaken by the author, on behalf of the American Anthropological Association, to explore the issues that are involved in the relationship between anthropologists and those agencies, both governmental and private, that sponsor their research. This study is an outcome of the Camelot affair which raised many important questions that bear upon the work of the anthropologist in foreign areas. This book is therefore mainly concerned with the ethics of the behaviour of American anthropologists working abroad, their relationship with social scientists and governments in 'host countries', and their relationship with the US government.

ENCEL, S., National Policies for the Social Sciences, *Social Science Information* **VII**, No. 3, pp. 201–7, June 1968.

The importance of the study of social science is because of the increasing rate of change of society. The author lists eight areas where this is particularly true and adds the international problem of the differences in the developed and non-developed countries; discusses the various forms of organization of research; lists six headings under which natural science policy may be discussed; these can also be used for social science policy.

(i) level of public support for R & D
(ii) allocation of resources between various institutions
(iii) scope and organization of government research activities
(iv) encouragement of research in particular fields
(v) application of scientific results in industry, medicine, etc.
(vi) manpower and education.

BRADFORD, B. HUDSON and PAGE, HOWARD, E., The Behavioral Sciences: Challenge and Partial Response, *American Behavioral Scientist* **6**, No. 8, pp. 3–7, 1963.

The authors point to the growing awareness of the potential of social science. They feel that there should be a new orientation towards research; the tools of the relevant disciplines should be brought together to solve the problems of society. Behavioural scientists should contribute not only to the understanding of the social processes but also to its control. They seem, however, to lack the self-confidence to press this home. This comes partly from the lack of support that has been shown by government and the universities, but the authors feel that the professional associations do not do enough to encourage their members, e.g. they should assume responsibility for the exchange of information with federal agencies and also for the effective transmittal of information to their members. The authors also feel that it is up to the professional associations to ensure that there is sufficient supply of graduates in each discipline to supply the demand; they should also know the areas where research is most needed. If the professional associations do not plan for the development of their disciplines, plans will be placed before them which they will be expected to follow.

REYNAUD, J. D., Une Politique des sciences sociales, *Revue française de sociologie* **6**, pp. 228–33, April–June 1965.

The author advocates the need in France for more extensive knowledge regarding the organization and social functions of social science research as a prerequisite to the formulation of policies for developing the social sciences.

2.1 Design of Institutions for Social Science Research and Training

CHERNS, A. B., *et al.*, Organization of Research, *Social Science Information* **6**, No. 4, pp. 224–47, August 1967.

These short articles are a reply to H. Friis's paper (pp. 215–25 above). Some are concerned with the situation in specific countries or institutes, but generally they attempt to answer the question 'what kind of research in what kind of organization?' using such criteria as the nature of the research (applied or basic), the need to build theory, the need to train researchers, the purposes of the research, the use of the research, and the need for interdisciplinary research.

CHOMBART DE LAUWE, P. H., MENDRAS, H., TOURAINE, A., Sociologie du travail sociologique, *Sociologie du travail* **7** (3), pp. 273–94, July–September 1965.

These papers, delivered at a meeting of the Société française de sociologie, have as a common theme the problem of reconciling the needs of empirical social research, such as team-work, division of labour, and careers specialized in the conduct of large-scale research, with traditional structures for support of research and the training of researchers.

FRIIS, HENNING, Division of Work between Research in Universities, Independent Institutes, and Government Departments, *Social Science Information* **5**, No. 1, pp. 5–11, March 1966.

This points to the work being undertaken in Scandinavia and Ireland to establish effective centres for applied research. Discusses necessary characteristics of organizations for applied research and three organizational ways of meeting these requirements: (a) individual policy bodies; (b) universities; and (c) independent multipurpose institutes.

KOROVIN, E. A., The Academy of Science of the USSR, *UNESCO Reports and Papers on Social Science*, No. 18, UNESCO, Paris, 1963.

In the USSR all research is planned at state level. The Academy of Science of the USSR is the supreme scientific organization responsible for research. In the Academy there are four divisions devoted to the humanities and history, to economics, to philosophy and law, and to linguistics. Each division is responsible for the identification and promotion of new trends, research activities on the most important problems, the organization of scientific discussions and meetings, the co-ordination of research work with other organizations, and international relations. A work plan is drawn up by each division and a section called 'organization of work on the problem' then assigns the given problems to the various institutes. These research institutes are the basic unit of research. They take part in the long-term plan for the national economy and culture, either by presenting to government bodies their recommendations or by direct participation in the activities of government planning organizations. The scientific council of the research institute discusses the research work, its procedure, and its publications, and organizes conferences and discussions. The problems of manpower are dealt with by the long-term plans, which include numbers of postgraduate scholarships, etc. The establishment of a permanent link between science and practical work is the most important principle of Soviet science. This work includes descriptions of the most important areas of research, and addresses of the institutes.

LAZARSFELD, P. F., Observations on the Organization of Empirical Social Research in the US, *Social Science Information* **1**, No. 1, pp. 3–37, 1961.

The rapid expansion of empirical work in the social sciences and the institutional forms this takes is one of the major innovations in higher education in the twentieth century. The author distinguishes four phases in this development: in the twenties the study of the communities in order to learn more about their social problems; in the thirties a concern for data rather than problems; post-war, experiments in attitudes and communications. In the fifties creation of organized social science research centres with teams rather than individuals. He discusses a survey carried out of 94 universities, 61 of which have clearcut organizational structures for social science research. The remaining 33, although they award higher degrees, have no formal research organization. Various characteristics of the units are examined – specialization of research topic, relationship with teaching departments, the role of the directors, the units as a service function, problems of training, career structures, financing, and choice of research topics.

ROSSI, P. H., Researchers, Scholars, and Policy-Makers: the Politics of Large-scale Research, *Daedalus*, No. 4, pp. 1142–61, 1964.

The author is interested in the growth of research centres within the university environment. These grew up partly as a means of eliminating the tensions between research and teaching in a university by separating them. In the social sciences the development of sample surveys as one of the main research techniques and the skills and time required for this give impetus for the growth of separate social science research centres. He discusses the various relationships between these centres and academic departments; the *ad hoc* finance in these centres affects the kind of research that is done and the researchers who will do it – little can be done by an individual researcher and often donors of money control what research is done; therefore much research is applied.

SCHAFF, ADAM, The Social Science Activities of the Eastern European Academies of Science, *UNESCO Reports and Papers on Social Science*, No. 18, UNESCO, Paris, 1963.

This describes the functions and organization of Eastern European Academies of Science which are a unique combination of 'corporations' of elected academies (similar to the Royal Society), research institutes, and bodies responsible for the organization, planning, and co-ordination of research on a national scale. The basic research unit of the academy is the institute, which is in turn divided into sectors. The academies also have national seminars, which bring together specialists in a particular field, primarily to co-ordinate their work but also to conduct joint research. Some institutes also have scientific councils whose task is the overall development of the disciplines, the co-ordination and planning of the research, and ensuring liaison between research and its practical application. The institutes issue periodicals and other publications and are responsible for the training of young scientists. The creation of independent research institutes may weaken the institutes of higher education, as the former will attract the best research workers, while the latter will still need to combine research with teaching. The work of the research institutes is conducted in accordance with a long-term plan covering a general theme and then broken down into individual research projects. It includes chapters on the academies of science in Bulgaria, Czechoslovakia, Hungary, Poland, Rumania, and Jugoslavia.

TIMLIN, M., FAUCHER, ALBERT, *The Social Sciences in Canada*, SSRCC, Ottawa, 136 pp., 1968.

The writers believe that the reason for the weakness in the social sciences in Canada and for the fact that they have fallen behind other nations lies in the institutional structure and in a lack of finance. They discuss the functions and history of the SSRCC and the Canada Council and where they feel these have failed in their function. Also examines the SSRCs of America and Holland, covering their overall philosophy, their conference and committee system, and their grants and fellowship policy. The authors make recommendations for the reconstruction of the institutions in Canada based on these two studies, suggesting that the SSRCC should be revitalized with as its central function the role of catalysing agency, planning and encouraging all aspects of social science research but not being responsible for subsidizing the actual process of the research. The second main function of such a body would be to disseminate information, register research projects, and keep abreast of new methodologies. The Canada Council should be split into the Canada Council for the Humanities and Social Sciences and the Canada Council for the Fine and Performing Arts. Its main functions would be to award grants and fellowships, to help professional associations and journals, to finance seminars, etc., and to help the SSRCC in its information function. The authors feel that the operations of the SSRCC should be financed from government on a continuing basis, although this need not necessarily be so for every research project that it may initiate.

US Senate Sub-Committee on Government Research, National Foundation for Social Sciences, Parts I–III, Hearings on S.836, US Government Printing Office, Washington, DC, 1967.

With Chairman Fred R. Harris, one of the most vigorous supporters of social science in Congress, doing most of the questioning, an array of government officialdom, science officialdom, and academic notables offer statements, testimony, and exhibits in hearings on the bill to establish a national foundation for the social sciences, 'in order to promote research and scholarship in such sciences'. The post–Project Camelot controversies set the stage for much of the discussion, but it ranges extensively through matters affecting the organization, financing, and uses of the social sciences.

VIET, J., *Les Sciences de l'homme en France, tendances et organisation de la recherche,* International Social Science Council Publications No. 7, Mouton, Paris, 1966.

Chapter VI contains an overview of organizational structures for the conduct and support of social science research in France.

2.2 The Financing of Social Science Research and Teaching

BIDERMANN, A. D., CRAWFORD, E. T., *The Political Economies of Social Research: Sociology*, Bureau of Social Science Research, Washington, DC, 106 pp., 1968.

Sociology grew up primarily in a university setting, though it was more knowledge producing than knowledge imparting; being relatively pure it stayed relatively poor. In the period up to the depression foundations provided the majority of the money for research, but sociology had still not established any legitimation for economic support. The crisis situation created by the New Deal and the war brought a consensus of values that enabled social scientists and government to work together, e.g. federal support for universities, research in military offices, 'in-house' research. During the period of the cold war social scientists have gained government support mainly through military offices, with the exception of health. The easing of the cold war, Project Camelot, and lack of sympathy with the Viet Nam war have led social scientists away from military research. But at present sociology has grown because of the government interest in problem areas, e.g. poverty, urban renewal, etc.

BIDERMANN, A. D., CRAWFORD, E. T., Paper Money: Trends of Research Sponsorship in American Sociology Journals, *Social Science Information* **9**, No. 1, pp. 51–77, 1970.

Data on extent and types of acknowledged sponsorship were obtained for all articles published in four American sociology journals for the years 1950 to 1968. Using this data, the authors examine the validity of some frequently voiced apprehensions regarding the impact of federal funds on published sociology.

CLARK, S. D., The Support of Social Science Research in Canada, *Canadian Journal of Economics and Political Science* **24** (No. 2), pp. 141–51, 1958.

In this article, which draws on a report prepared for the Social Science Research Council of Canada, the author points out that despite increases in financial resources brought about by the establishment of the Canada Council and a Ford Foundation grant to the SSRCC, certain restrictions, particularly the heavy teaching loads, still limit the amount and quality of social science research carried out in Canadian universities.

CUISENIER, J., La Sociologie et ses applications: recherche sur programme et recherche sur contract, *Revue française de sociologie* **7**, pp. 361–80, Juillet–Septembre 1966.

The interaction between sociological enterprise in France and its significant publics is presented as a problem of making the supply of sociological knowledge products meet existing demands. Contract and programme financing are viewed as two alternative means of regulating this 'market'. This article was presented as a talk delivered to the Société française de sociologie, followed by a discussion.

ELLIS, W., The Federal Government in Behavioral Science Fields, Methods and Funds, *American Behavioral Scientist* 7, No. 9, pp. 3–24, May 1964.

This article, although now rather outdated, is one of the most comprehensive attempts to analyse the role of the American government in supporting social science. It starts with a summary of the history of government social science relations. It has detailed information of the support for social science research by various government departments, broken down into fields of study. The report also carries figures of social science manpower employed by the federal government.

GORDON, G., PARELIUS, ANN, & MARQUIS, SUE, Public versus private support of science, *American Behavioral Scientist* 10, No. 9, pp. 29–31, 1967.

This article considers some of the pros and cons for public and private research support in terms of innovativeness, freedom of researchers, etc., but among scientists themselves no clear pattern emerges. Reports a survey of various sources of finance in the field of medical sociology and finds that over all federal money was used in more innovative research than private support, but this is exaggerated by the fact that private research in a state or local level scores very low on the innovative scale.

JOHNSON, H. G., The Social Sciences in the Age of Opulence, *Canadian Journal of Economics and Political Science* 32, No. 4, pp. 423–42, November 1966.

This is the presidential address given at the thirty-eighth annual meeting of the Canadian Political Science Association. It discusses problems resulting from the increased material benefits that accrue to social scientists in a situation of an expanding system of higher education and growth in demand for applied research and advisory services. It includes data on salaries of Canadian political scientists and economists in academic and government employment.

DE JOUVENEL, BERTRAND, Situation des sciences sociales aux États-Unis (The State of the social sciences in the United States), *Analyse et Prévision* 5, pp. 319–36, May 1968.

A study of the state of the social sciences in the United States, with emphasis on the financing based on an examination of the relevant literature. Social sciences accounted for 31 per cent of the doctorates granted in 1958–62 and 30 per cent in 1962. The National Science Foundation has a narrower definition of social sciences than that of A. M. Cartter, whose statistics are quoted above; it excludes business, education, law, library science, and social science. A congressional inquiry in 1964 found that government support of social science research amounted that year to $197 million out of $4,464 million spent on science. Social sciences have been reduced to an ancillary position, especially in the determination of scientific policies. However, there are large discrepancies in the estimates of government money spent on the social sciences. The concept of social sciences as 'behavioural' poses the threat of a divorce from the traditional humanities, but this threat has been minimized by the tie-up between government financing of social science research and the political aims of the Great Society.

National Science Foundation, *Scientific Activities at Universities and Colleges*, Washington, DC, Government Printing Office, XIV, 96 pp., 1964.

Based on a survey conducted in 1964, this report gives data on current direct and capital expenditures for research and instruction in the social sciences at American universities and colleges.

National Science Foundation, *Federal Funds for Research Development and Other Scientific Activities*, XVII (FY 1967, 1968, 1969), US Government Printing Office, Washington, DC, 1968.

Issued annually, this publication provides statistical data on the amount of funds obligated by government agencies for research in the several social science disciplines, the types of institutions receiving funds, and the amount of funds obligated for collection of scientific data regarding social phenomena.

2.3 Manpower Questions

CARTER, M. P., Report on the Survey of Sociological Research in Britain, *Sociological Review* **16**, No. 1, pp. 5–40, March 1968.

Report of a questionnaire sent to 1000 members of the BSA – 416 replies were received. The analysis of these gives data on age qualifications, and type of post. Also has information on research work past, present, and future – how it is financed, what are the main subjects of interest, and what are the main handicaps to research; also suggests growth points and neglected areas.

GROENMANN, S., KÖNIG, R., CLAESSENS, D., Die Berufsmöglichkeiten des Soziologen (The occupational opportunities of sociologists), *Kölner Zeitschrift für Soziologie und Sozialpsychologie* 14, pp. 271–321, 1962.

Proceedings of one of the sessions at a meeting of the Deutsche Gesell schaft für Soziologie in Tübingen in 1961. Groenmann discusses careers of sociologists in non-university employment with particular reference to the Dutch situation. König reports data from a survey of the education of sociologists at the University of Köln, 1950–60, and their subsequent employment experiences. Claessens summarizes the subsequent discussion.

HALL, MICHAEL, Research vs. Industry, *Higher Education Review*, pp. 28–44, spring, 1969.

Although this article is concerned with the supply of scientists and engineers, the more general topic of the lack of regulation between the output from universities and the demand for industry is of concern to manpower problems in general. There is no longer any automatic way of relating demand and supply; university expansion has not reflected the clearly expressed demand for certain types of manpower. As the several government reports on qualified manpower have all agreed, this situation is too anomalous to be left as it is.

HOPPER, JANICE H., Preliminary Report on Salaries and Selected Characteristics of Sociologists in the 1966 National Science Foundation Register of Scientific and Technical Personnel, *American Sociologist* 2, pp. 151–4, August 1967.

This article contains much data on number of degrees, primary work activity, employer, salary, and geographic distribution of American sociologists. It compares figures for 1964 and 1966, and concludes there is no substantial difference.

National Science Foundation, The Structure of Economists' Employment and Salaries, 1964, *American Economic Review* 4, No. 4, part 2 supplement, December 1965.

This contains data on economists, including age, work, degree, subject of interest, sex, salary, and employer; it includes various classifications to give very full coverage of data.

SCHLOTTMAN, U., Soziologen im Beruf: Zur beruflichen Situation der Absolventen eines soziologischen Studiums in Deutschland – erster Bericht über eine Untersuchung (Sociologists in the Profession: the Professional Situation of Those having finished their Sociological Studies in Germany – first report of survey), *Kölner Zeitschrift für Soziologie und Sozialpsychologie* 20, No. 3, pp. 572–97, September 1968.

A survey of university graduates who have received degrees since 1958, in which sociology figures as a major or minor subject (717 out of a universe of 815 individuals), which was undertaken for the purpose of obtaining information concerning types of organizations employing sociology graduates, types of positions held, earning patterns, and chances of promotion. The data enables the author to draw some tentative conclusions concerning the degree of professionalization in German sociology.

SCOTT, A., The Recruitment and Migration of Canadian Social Scientists, *Canadian Journal of Economics and Political Science* **33**, No. 4. pp. 495–508, November 1967.

This is a discussion of university staffing and recruitment problems in economics and political science brought about by increased undergraduate enrolment. The migration and importation of staffs to and from the US is given special consideration.

US Department of Commerce Bureau of Census, *The Postal Censal Survey, Characteristics of America's Engineers and Scientists, 1960 and 1962,* Government Printing Office, Washington, DC, Vol. VI, 73 pp. (Technical Paper No. 21), 1960.

In this survey, conducted in 1962, of a sample of occupational groups drawn from the population enumerated in the 1960 census, social scientists figure alongside engineers, physical scientists, biological scientists, and mathematicians. It provides information on the numbers, sex, and age of social scientists in the US, on their work activities and employing institutions, as well as on their educational preparation.

2.4 Documents Relating to the Formulation of Social Science Policies in Different Countries

FRIIS, H., Development of Social Research in Ireland, *Institute of Public Administration*, Dublin, 1965.

An examination of the institutional framework for social research in Ireland and recommendations for the establishment of an Institute of Social Research, including details of required finance, staffing, and links with established bodies such as the universities.

LORD HEYWORTH (chairman), *Report of the Committee on Social Studies,* Cmnd. 2660, HMSO, 100 pp., 1965.

'. . . to review the research at present being done in the field of social science in Government Departments, Universities and other institutions and to advise whether changes are needed in the arrangements for supporting and co-ordinating this research.' The main recommendation of the report is the formation of a Social Science Research Council.

NAS/SSRC Behavioral and Social Science Survey Committee (BASS), *The Behavioral and Social Sciences: Outlook and Needs*, National Academy of Sciences, 1969.

This report is the result of a survey carried out by the BASS Committee, which was set up in 1966 to look at the 'present status and future needs of the component disciplines and their joint research activities'. Because the organization of the social sciences is still around the basic disciplines, separate survey reports of the disciplines will also be published. The survey had two main tasks: to assess the nature of the behavioural and social science enterprise in terms of its past growth, present size and anticipated development; and to suggest ways in which these sciences might contribute to both basic understanding of human behaviour and effective social planning and policy-making. Much of the report is concerned with this first task of showing how the social sciences are financed and organized and contains some very useful statistics. The committee feels that the present organization of university departments is too strongly directed along disciplinary lines to be effective in solving social problems – they suggest the establishment of graduate schools of applied behavioural science. Many of the recommendations concerning the relationship of the federal government and social science are similar to those put forward in the NAS report *The Behavioral Sciences and the Federal Government*, e.g. representation on the President's Science Advisory Committee and the Office of Science and Technology, and the increase of funds for social science from federal sources. This report lays emphasis on social indicators and their role in the development of a social report and the eventual establishment of a council of social advisers. The committee also suggest the creation of a 'National Data System' to centralize statistics and in this context discusses the problem of privacy and ethics.

EULAU, HEINZ, MARCH, JAMES G. (eds.), *Political Science*, Prentice-Hall, Englewood Cliffs, N.J., vii, 148 pp., 1969.

SMELSER, NEIL J., DAVIS, JAMES A. (eds.), *Sociology*, Prentice-Hall, Englewood Cliffs, N.J., ix, 178 pp., 1969.

OECD, *The Social Sciences and the Policies of Governments*, OECD, Paris, 102 pp., 1966.

This considers the development of the social sciences in OECD-member countries which are discussed under such headings as 'Fundamental and applied research', 'Social sciences and policy-makers', 'Organization of research', and 'The social functions of social sciences'. The last chapter sets forth some guidelines to help governments formulate national social science policies. It includes data on amount and sources of support for social science research in selected countries.

Tavistock Institute, *Social Research and a National Policy for Science*, Tavistock Publications, London, Pamphlet No. 7, 44 pp., 1964.

This study of social science policy outlines questions of co-ordination and support of social science research in Great Britain with reference to three types of research organizations (those located in user-organizations, in university departments, and in special purpose research institutes). It includes estimates of the future rate of growth of the social sciences and the funds needed to sustain this growth.

2.5 Types of Decisions Affecting Social Science Policies

Congress and Social Science, *American Psychologist*, pp. 877–1041, November 1967.

'In years to come, the 90th Congress opening in 1967, may be viewed as the place and time of the take-off point for the underdeveloped social and behavioral sciences' (Introduction). The issue includes testimony before the senate sub-committee on government research of the Committee on Government Operations relating to a proposed National Foundation for the Social Sciences and on the 'Full Opportunity and Social Accounting Act of 1967'.

BREZINA, DENNIS W., The Congressional Debate on the Social Sciences in 1968, Staff Discussion Paper 400, *Program of Policy Studies in Science and Technology*, George Washington University, Washington, D.C., 1968.

The author discusses the debates that took place in congress mainly in senate during 1968 that related to the social sciences. Since the Camelot affair, and with the bill by Senator Harris to establish a NSSF, the social sciences have come out from under the protective umbrella of the natural sciences, at least in public debate. They still have not formed a strong political base for themselves; they have no agency equivalent to the NSF (for the natural sciences), and they have little representation on congressional science advisory bodies. Until the social sciences can establish such a base they are going to be open to the sort of political buffeting reported in this paper, and they are therefore unable to reach their full potential.

3. THE USE OF THE SOCIAL SCIENCES IN POLICY OR PLANNING

3.0 General writings
3.1 Alternative conceptions of the process of utilization
3.2 Use of social science research in public policy-making
3.3 Use of social science research in industry

3.0 General Writings

DROR, YEHEZKEL, Some Normative Implications of a Systems View of Policy-making, Rand Corporation (P3991–1), Santa Monica, California, 22 pp., February 1969.

The author suggests the use of a normative systems approach to analyse the operation of the policy-making process and to make suggestions for improving this process. Because public policy-making is the interaction of a large number of various components, similar changes in output can be achieved through many alternative changes in the components – improvements must reach a critical mass in order to influence the aggregate output of the system. Although efforts are being made to improve the policy-making processes, these do not take account of the total complex system and often do not reach the critical mass and are, therefore, ineffectual.

LAZARSFELD, PAUL, SEWELL, WILLIAM, & WILENSKY, HAROLD (eds.), *The Uses of Sociology*, Basic Books, New York, 901 pp., 1967.

The origin of this volume was the American Sociological Association Annual Meeting in 1962 which was devoted to the topic 'The Uses of Sociology'. It contains papers by more than 40 present-day sociologists on the uses of sociology for different social purposes and in different institutional contexts. The introduction by Lazarsfeld suggests typologies for the problems to which sociology is applied and the roles of applied sociologists.

LYONS, GENE, *The Uneasy Partnership*, Russell Sage Foundation, New York, 1969.

The book provides a comprehensive account of the social sciences within the federal government in the twentieth century. The author suggests three main reasons for the steady growth of social science programmes: (a) the growth of the federal government and its increased influence on economic and social affairs; (b) the development of the social sciences, both in collecting and analysing data and in developing theories based on empirical evidence; (c) improvements in administrative management.

The author argues strongly for strengthening the role of the social sciences in the federal government, and for creating a central organization for developing policies for the social sciences.

NSF (Special Commission on the Social Sciences of the National Science Board), Knowledge into Action: Improving the Nation's Use of the Social Sciences, US Government Printing Office, Washington, D.C., 1969.

The Special Commission on the Social Sciences established by the

National Science Board in 1968 was charged with making recommendations for increasing the useful application of the social sciences in the solution of contemporary social problems. The Commission, moreover, believes that the nation is missing crucial opportunities to utilize fully social science knowledge and skills in the formulation, evaluation, and execution of policies for achieving desired social goals. The Commission points to four main obstacles to the utilization of social science knowledge:

(i) there is no institution or agency to note the knowledge and act on it
(ii) often social science can only provide descriptions or precedents, but not solutions, and hence the knowledge is rejected
(iii) it may threaten the *status quo*
(iv) others reject the knowledge even when they agree with it because the resources demanded to implement it are too great.

Although the Commission is interested in increasing the use of existing knowledge, they fully recognize the need for continued support for objective social research.

The Commission looks at the relationship that has existed between social science and five other groups – the professions, the federal government, business and labour, community organizations, and the public – and recommends ways in which these relationships may be strengthened. The Commission also looks at the need for special problem research institutes.

3.1 Alternative Conceptions of the Process of Utilization

ARCHIBALD, KATHLEEN, The Utilization of Social Research and Policy Analysis, unpublished thesis, George Washington University, Washington, D.C., 456 pp., 1968.

Based in part on the existing literature, in part on interviews with government officials and policy-oriented scholars, this thesis discusses alternative role orientations of policy-oriented social scientists, with particular reference to international security. The three alternative orientations to the applied role are labelled the *academic*, the *clinical*, and the *strategic*. Utilization of the social sciences in policy formulation is regarded as a relatively unstructured exchange process between members of different social systems. The historical and institutional contexts of social research and policy analysis are set forth in two appendices entitled 'Federal Interest and Investment in Social Science' and 'Social Science and International Security'.

The first appendix was reprinted in Research and Technical Programs Sub-Committee, Committee on Government Operations, US House of Representatives: The Use of Social Research in Federal Domestic Programs, Part I, 90th Congress, 1st Session, pp. 314–40, 1967.

CHERNS, A. B., The Use of the Social Sciences, *Human Relations* **21**, No. 4, November 1968.

This attempts to answer five questions: (i) why study the social sciences? (ii) why study them in a university of technology? (iii) what is the use of all the research that is done? (iv) why is it not more useful? (v) what do we intend to do about it? The author discusses the utilization and non-utilization of social science research giving various examples from India, Israel, and Australia.

CHERNS, A. B., Social Research and its Diffusion, *Human Relations* **22**, No. 3, pp. 209–18, 1969.

Much of the failure to use social research lies in a misconception of the processes whereby research is translated into action. Part of this misconception lies in the distinction between pure and applied, theoretical and empirical research. The author offers an alternative classification: (i) pure basic research; (ii) basic objective research; (iii) operational research; (iv) action research.

Illustrations are given of various research projects that fit into these categories. From these illustrations it can be seen that as we pass from basic pure research to action research utilization is more likely, but the generality of the results is diminished. We also find that the diffusion channels are different.

The main problem would therefore seem to be the improvement of the research action diffusion channel to enable greater utility of results. Although the author gives no solution to this, he points to the research being done in this area at the Centre for the Utilization of Social Science Research at Loughborough University.

DROR, Y., *Public Policy-Making Re-Examined*, Chandler, San Francisco, 1968.

This book is concerned with a theoretical approach to the problems of public policy-making, centred on the thesis that there is a significant gap between the ways individuals and institutions make policy, and the available knowledge on how policies can best be made. Such policies about policies he terms 'meta-policy-making'.

The author claims that it is possible to develop a policy science that will improve the quality of public policy-making and then deals vigorously and comprehensively with the problems of the evaluation of public policy-making, the construction of an optimal model, and the major changes needed (in structure, knowledge, and personnel, in particular). Useful appendices include a long bibliography essay and several tabular presentations of arguments in the text.

HEISKANEN, VERONICA STOLTE, Uses of Sociology: A Case Study of Commissioned Research in Finland, *Social Science Information* **8**, No. 3, pp. 87–98, 1969.

This article starts by showing how two sets of criteria may affect society's support of sciences: internal criteria on degree of competence in the field; external criteria on evaluation of how far science illuminates other fields or furthers technological or social goals. However, among the academic social science community there seems to be a fear of being non-academic if they deal with solely practical problems. There is no recognized profession of applied social scientists and most work of this nature is still done as a 'non-profit-making' venture by academics or research institutions. The article is concerned with the use of the results of commissioned research and reports the research of a survey of 20 such projects undertaken in Finland. It analyses the projects by types of client and form of research and then studies how the results were utilized.

It relates the clients' satisfaction with the research to whether policy recommendations were included and whether the research findings are used. A typology of the research based on these criteria does not give a very clear picture. The author feels this is due to the lack of appropriate organization of applied research and of the attitude of the professional community towards it. She also feels strongly the need for further research along the lines of her small survey so that more evidence may be gathered about the utilization of research findings.

HOROWITZ, IRVING LOUIS, Social Science and Public Policy: Some Implications of Modern Research, in *The Rise and Fall of Project Camelot*, I. L. Horowitz (ed.), MIT Press, Cambridge, Mass., pp. 339–76, 1967.

Part I classifies three kinds of political systems and the role of the social sciences in them:

(i) in a command society policy dictates both the character and activities of the social sciences which then lose control over both the instruments and purposes of research
(ii) in a welfare system, policy and social science interact but without any sense of tension or contradiction between scientific propositions and the therapeutic orientations
(iii) in a laissez-faire system, the social sciences tend to be independent and autonomous of political policy.

Part II discusses the problem of the norm of secrecy as applied by policy-makers and how this affects their relations with social scientists.

Part III considers the university bureaucracies and value systems and the author suggests it is worth considering the degree to which the strain between social scientific activities and policy-making activities ought to be viewed as a conflict of rules between feudal, university-based, and modern state-based institutions.

Part IV considers whether the policy-maker and the social scientist should remain separate entities – the classic rationale for a tighter linkage is a higher sense of responsibility for the social scientist and a greater degree of training for the policy-oriented personnel, but the author feels the realities of the situation are such that the utility of the social sciences to policy-making bodies depends upon some maintenance of the separation of the social sciences from the policy situation.

LIPPITT, R., The Use of Social Research to Improve Social Practise, *American Journal of Orthopsychiatry* 35, No. 4, pp. 663–9, July 1965.

This discusses some of the experiences of the staff of the Center for Research on Utilization of Scientific Knowledge, and summarizes six models of the research utilization process, illustrating these from research projects the Center has undertaken. Briefly these models are: (i) derivation of action designs from relevant research findings; (ii) the adoption of experimentally tested models of practice; (iii) diffusion between practitioners; (iv) diagnostic team with feedback; (v) internal action-research process; (vi) the training of consumers to be open to the use of science. A number of differences exist between research utilization in the social sciences and in the applied biological and physical sciences. The research utilization function of the staff of the Center is to act as linking agents at various points in the flow of research use. This has implications for the training of utilization agents.

LOMPE, KLAUS, The Role of the Social Scientist in the Processes of Policy-Making, *Social Science Information* 7, No. 6, pp. 159–75, 1968.

The author attempts to answer the following questions:

(i) Should social scientists play an advisory role in politics?
(ii) Will they be allowed to play this role?
(iii) Are social scientists capable of giving advice in politics?
(iv) If so, what kind of advice should be given?
(v) How is the co-operation between scientists and politicians to be organized?

Three models that describe the complex relationship between science and politics are discussed – these are the 'technocratic', the 'decisionistic', and the 'pragmatist'.

For many reasons, there has been growing dissatisfaction with the first two models for relating social science to policy-making and the author sees the pragmatist model as an alternative – the functional separation of the roles of the politician and adviser is replaced by a critical dialogue – where value judgements, goals, and empirical facts can be brought together. We can regard this type of relationship as based on long-term co-operation between scientists, politicians, and civil servants where all participants learn from one another.

TRIST, E. L., *The Professional Facilitation of Planned Change in Organizations*, 17th International Congress of Applied Psychology, Swets and Zeitlinger, Amsterdam, August 1968.

The rapid rate at which change is now taking place has posed new problems for organizations and the individuals within them. The author suggests that planned organizational change can best be achieved by coupling the resources of the social sciences with the competences already in the organization, establishing a collaborative action-research-type relationship. Although there is joint responsibility for bringing about the change towards agreed ends, the responsibility for actually introducing any change must remain with the client. It is important that evaluation of what happens should be continuously made, thereby increasing the social knowledge within the organization and also the knowledge of the scientific community. The author gives a history of this sort of collaborative research relationship and how it has developed since the war.

ZETTERBERG, H., The Practical Uses of Sociological Knowledge, *Acta Sociologica* 7, No. 2, pp. 57–71, 1964.

The author discusses five alternative role orientations through which social scientists can put their knowledge products to use. Illustrative problems are given for each alternative.

3.2 The Use of Social Science Research in Public Policy-Making

CRAWFORD, E., BIDERMANN, A. D. (eds.), *Social Scientist and International Affairs*, John Wiley, New York, 1969.

The main theme of this book is the relationship between social scientists and government with special reference to the area of international affairs. The purpose of the editors in producing this book is to show the need for and validity of a sociology of social science – social science has now grown to be 'big science' and as such we can talk about the institution of social science. Hence it can be studied using conceptual frameworks similar to those used by sociologists in their study of other institutions.

As this is a collection of reprints covering the whole of the post-war period, there is nothing new in what is said, but the editors have used lengthy introductory chapters to bring these readings together under four main sections:

(i) perspectives on the social roles of the social sciences
(ii) the social organization of policy-oriented social science
(iii) the affairs of social scientists with the affairs of state
(iv) the functions of policy-oriented social science.

This book also contains a comprehensive annotated bibliography.

DAS, R., Action Research and its Importance in an Underdeveloped Economy, Planning Research and Action Institute, Lucknow, India, pp. ii–74, 1963.

Describes the work of the Planning Research and Action Institute in transmitting knowledge concerning socioeconomic development to rural populations in the state of Uttar Pradesh in Northern India.

FONDATION ROYAUMONT, *Le psychosociologie dans la cité: l'école, l'hôpital, l'entreprise, le syndicat*, Éditions de l'Épi, Paris, 334 pp., 1967.

Proceedings of a conference examining the interaction between social psychologists and diverse social institutions, with particular emphasis on their roles as social practitioners and reformers.

HOROWITZ, IRVING LOUIS, The Academy and the Polity: Interaction between Social Scientists and Federal Administrators, *Journal of Applied Behavioral Science* 5, No. 3, pp. 309–35, September 1969.

In this paper the author considers how academics view politicians and how politicians view academics, and notes that the difficulties and problems involved in this relationship are perceived differently by the two parties. The author then shows how relations between the two sectors have changed over the period since the war, e.g. the interdisciplinary 'policy sciences' approach of Laswell, the 'hand maiden approach' where social scientists were to supply the knowledge and make the politicians more effective, the selective participation approach where there would be equality and parity between the social scientists and administrators but this largely through unplanned interchanges. He notes that forms of non-participation are becoming more important, mainly as a reaction to the contract state and fears about the autonomy of the science. This non-participation has in some areas turned to active opposition, mainly because of the political and ideological climate that now prevails.

HOROWITZ, IRVING LOUIS (ed.), *The Rise and Fall of Project Camelot: Studies in the Relationship between Social Science and Practical Politics*, MIT Press, Cambridge, Mass., 385 pp., 1967.

The book examines the 'Camelot Affair' under five different headings and from five different perspectives. These are: the setting of the 'Project

Camelot'; its design and purposes; the academic response to its cancellation; the political response; and, the general implications of the 'Camelot Affair'. Included are articles by I. L. Horowitz, R. Boguslaw, J. Galtung, and R. A. Nisbet.

IATRIDIS, D., Social Scientists in Physical Development Planning: A Practitioner View-point, *International Social Science Journal* **18**, No. 4, pp. 515–38, 1966.

The potential contribution of members of different social science disciplines in teams engaging in planning rural-urban development is set forth for each phase of the planning process. The author also discusses ways of improving the effectiveness of social scientists in these teams.

LEAR, J., Public Policy and the Study of Man, *Saturday Review*, pp. 59–62, 7 September 1968.

This article points out a growing interest in what has been referred to as the 'fourth dimension' of government, which would be concerned with relating research to public policy. It quotes Dr Golovin of the OST as seeing the function of his fourth branch to be:

(a) to collect all the data necessary to continually track the state of the nation
(b) define potential problems suggested by the information
(c) develop alternate plans to cope with the problems
(d) evaluate ongoing projects in terms of real time and advise the people accordingly.

The article then goes on to review the report of the NAS/NRC report *The Behavioral Sciences and the Federal Government* in the light of the fourth dimension. One comment the article makes is that it expects any developments arising from the report to be slow in showing themselves as concrete outcomes. This is because, as the article points out, talk about the role of social science knowledge in policy-making has been taking place for over twelve years without much effect.

National Academy of Sciences/National Research Council, *The Behavioral Sciences and the Federal Government,* Publication No. 1680, NAS, 1968.

The purpose of this report is to examine how the knowledge and methods of the behavioural sciences can be brought to bear effectively on the programmes and policy processes of the federal government. The report discusses this under six headings: government's need for knowledge and information; lessons of experience; effective use of the behavioural sciences; behavioural science and international affairs; science policies and the behavioural sciences; development of the behavioural sciences. The report puts forward ten important recommendations. The first three are concerned with the conditions that the report feels are necessary for the effective use of behavioural science in government. The fourth recommendation concerns foreign area research. The fifth and sixth recommendations are concerned with international co-operation. The seventh and eighth are concerned with the position of the behavioural sciences as regards the present structure for science policy. The ninth is concerned with the role of the NSF as regards the behavioural sciences, their encouragement of basic research, and studying the future needs for development and use of the behavioural sciences. The tenth recommendation is for the establishment of an independent National Institute for Advance Research and Public Policy. This body would undertake continuing long-range analysis of national policies and serve as a forum for discussion on all aspects of knowledge of science and its application to the issues of society.

Research and Technical Programs Sub-Committee, US House of Representatives, The Use of Social Research in Federal Domestic Programs, US House of Representatives 90th Congress, Session 1, Parts I–IV, 1967.

A staff study by the committee, which makes extensive use of writings by social scientists and others on numerous aspects of the relationship of government agencies, primarily domestic ones and social science disciplines. The results of surveys conducted by committee staffs of federal social research programmes and of the attitudes of some scientists towards government support are included in Parts I and III respectively.

3.3 Use of Social Science Research in Industry

BARITZ, L., *Servants of Power: A History of Social Science in American Industry*, Wesleyan University Press, Middletown, Conn., 1960.

The author traces the development of the use of social sciences in American industry from the late nineteenth century to 1960, e.g. the development of human relations, the introduction of aptitude tests, etc. But the author maintains that the owners or managers of American industry have only introduced social benefits, increased participation by improved understanding of the workers because in this way they can have more efficient factories. Author feels that industrial social scientists are the servants of management and hence of power. They can only do research on what management wants and any recommendation will only be accepted if management hopes thereby to make some profit. Industrial social scientists have not developed a theoretical approach to the subject, but they face problems as they arise.

BENNIS, W. G., Behavioural Science and Planned Organizational Change, in *Operational Research and the Social Sciences*, J. Lawrence (ed.), Tavistock Publications, London, 1966.

The author discusses and compares Operational Research and Planned Change. Examines theories of change and their bases and in addition the characteristics of change agents and client systems, and suggests some conditions and qualifications surrounding planned change.

BROWN, R. K., Research and Consultancy in Industrial Enterprises, *Sociology* 1, No. 1, pp. 33–60, January 1967.

The four major contributions of the Tavistock Institute of Human Relations to industrial sociology reviewed in this article are: the development of an 'open sociotechnical systems' model of the industrial organization; the study of industrial work groups; the elaboration of ideas concerning management organization; and discussion of sources of resistance to change in organization. The limitations of these contributions stemming from research carried out as consultative work are discussed.

CHERNS, A. B., CLARK, P. A., A Role for the Social Scientists in Organization Design, OR & Behavioural Science Conference, London, December 1968, in G. Heald (ed.), *Approaches to the Study of Organizational Behaviour*, Tavistock Publications, London, 1970.

This paper is divided into two parts. The first describes the earlier stages in a research/consultancy project concerning the social and psychological aspects involved in the design of a new factory, reporting in particular the use of sociotechnical analysis and the working relationship developed between the researchers and the clients.

The second part identifies and discusses some of the problems that face social scientists as members of multidisciplinary groups when working in the relatively uncharted territory of organizational design.

DUNNETTE, M. D., BROWN, Z. M. Behavioural Science Research and the Conduct of Business, *Academy of Management Journal* 2, No. 2, 1968.

Increasingly businessmen are aware of relevant applications to industry of behavioural science research. This paper attempts to assess the impact of sociological and psychological research on business, its use, and relative value as accorded by researchers and executives. It reports on a study that pointed to the different dimensions social scientists and business executives considered important in research studies.

FERGUSON, LAWRENCE L., Social Scientists in the Plant, *Harvard Business Review* 42, pp. 133–43, 1964.

The article reports the experiences of the General Electric Company in setting up and operating the Behavioral Research Services. Examples are given of social science findings that have been utilized within the organization. Many of the examples concern psychological or social psychological work. A number of observations are made that relate to the use of social scientists and social science knowledge within organizations.

LUPTON, T., *Management and the Social Sciences*, Hutchinson, London, 1966.
Here the author discusses the various social sciences and their subject matter and describes some of the early theories about industrial organization. He summarizes some of the research carried out by social scientists in industry, their methods, and the knowledge of industrial organizations as social systems which is being accumulated. He considers more specifically what social science has to offer to the manager by referring to some practical problems, and outlines some current developments in the theory of organizations.

4. INTERNATIONAL COLLABORATION IN THE SOCIAL SCIENCES

HOCHFELD, J., Patterns of UNESCO's Social Science Programme, *International Social Science Journal* **18**, No. 4, pp. 569–88, 1966.
This is a very detailed and useful paper which discusses the place of the social sciences in the system of constitutional purposes and functions of UNESCO. It shows the changes in emphasis in the social science sector of UNESCO as the UN has changed, especially in membership, over the years; describes the recent reorganization and the splitting of the proposed budget for 1967/8.

MEYNAUD, JEAN, International Co-operation in the Field of the Social Sciences, *UNESCO Reports and Papers in the Social Sciences,* No. 13, UNESCO, Paris, 1961.
The author attempts to analyse the present situation of international bodies in the social sciences.
UNESCO was largely instrumental in creating the international association for each social scientific discipline that exists at present – also for the existing ISSC. Some of the problems, particularly in the social sciences, in establishing international bodies are due to differences in ideologies, but problems can also be caused by discipline boundaries and personality conflicts.
The working of international bodies has helped in the tremendous growth in the development of the social sciences in almost every country, and more particularly in international co-operation and interdisciplinary

co-operation, and has also made valuable contributions in the area of the application of social science and the creation of professional tools.

The work of these international bodies would be helped by: (i) clarification and re-assessment of aims; (ii) increases in financial resources; (iii) long-term planning; and (iv) improvement in the internal atmosphere of such bodies.

MARSHALL, T. H., International Co-operation in the Social Sciences, Paper in International Organizations in the Social Sciences, UNESCO, Paris, 1965.

This paper describes the history of international co-operation and the problems that have arisen; differences in culture; language; ideology; and the distance involved in travelling. It points to the role international and interdisciplinary bodies can play in developing the social sciences.

ROKKAN, S. The Development of Cross-cultural Comparative Research: A Review of Current Problems and Possibilities, *Social Science Information* 1, No. 3, pp. 21–38, 1962.

The author discusses the UNESCO programme resolution which authorizes the Director General to 'facilitate the study of basic theories and concepts as well as of methods and techniques in cross-cultural social science research and to publish or arrange for the publication of results'. The programme is elaborated as follows: role of UNESCO; role of ISSC; action to promote comparative survey research; a general programme of action to promote comparative research.

5. BIBLIOGRAPHIES

CRAWFORD, ELISABETH T. The Sociology of the Social Sciences: An International Bibliography, *Social Science Information* 9, No. 1, 1970 (continuing).

This is the first instalment of a bibliography in the sociology of social sciences to be published bi-annually in *Social Science Information*. The bibliography contains selected references to material dealing with the social, economic, and political organization of the social sciences in various countries. Apart from a section of general writings, there are four main topic headings, which are further subdivided. The main headings are: theory and method of the sociology of the social sciences; historical perspectives on the social sciences; the institutionalization of the social sciences; the economics of social science research and teaching.

FORD, JANET, & PLUMB, BARBARA, Bibliography on the Utilization of Social Science Knowledge with particular Reference to Planned Organizational Change, Part I, Centre for Utilization of Social Science Research, University of Technology, Loughborough, Leicestershire, 1970 (mimeographed).

The field covered concerns social science utilization within organizations, particularly industrial situations, but excluding governmental use of social science research. Of the many forms utilization can take, the focus is on the use of social science knowledge to devise and achieve planned organizational change.

Two main sources of material have been used: published accounts by practitioners and consultants of their experience in planned change, and reports by people studying the consultancy and planning of change processes from a research viewpoint.

The material is grouped under ten headings: antecedent factors; change agents; client systems; consultant/client relationship; diffusion of information; entry and exit procedures and problems; resistance to and failure of utilization; research into the process of utilization; models and ideal types of utilization; definitions, parameters, and competences of utilization and planned organizational change.

SINCLAIR, RUTH, Bibliography of Social Science Policy, Centre for Utilization of Social Science Research University of Technology, Loughborough, Vols. I–III, 1968–70 (mimeograph).

This bibliography is part of the project on social science policy, being carried out with the aid of a grant from the International Social Science Council, and covers a wide range of subjects all of which are related to the development and use of the social sciences, but are also interrelated and must be considered in the formation of any social science policy. There are six main headings (which are further subdivided): the functions and roles of the social sciences; conditions for effective research; how much and what kind of research; aspects of evaluation and application; international collaboration; the idea of a social science policy.

STRAUS, M. A., Bibliography: Sociology of Social Research. Unpublished bibliography prepared for sociology seminar, University of New Hampshire, Durham, N.H., 39 pp., 1967.

This bibliography list references to a wide range of US publications dealing with most aspects of the conduct and organization of social science research with particular emphasis on research in sociology. It covers the period 1930–67.

For Product Safety Concerns and Information please contact our EU
representative GPSR@taylorandfrancis.com
Taylor & Francis Verlag GmbH, Kaufingerstraße 24, 80331 München, Germany

www.ingramcontent.com/pod-product-compliance
Ingram Content Group UK Ltd.
Pitfield, Milton Keynes, MK11 3LW, UK
UKHW022111190926
475702UK00013B/1377
9780415869072